VACCINES

VACCINES
WHAT YOU
SHOULD KNOW
THIRD EDITION

Paul A. Offit, M.D.

&

Louis M. Bell, M.D.

WILEY

John Wiley & Sons, Inc.

Published by John Wiley & Sons, Inc., Hoboken, New Jersey
Published simultaneously in Canada

For general information about our other products and services, please contact our Customer Care Department within the United States at (800) 762-2974, outside the United States at (317) 572-3993 or fax (317) 572-4002.

Wiley also publishes its books in a variety of electronic formats. Some content that appears in print may not be available in electronic books. For more information about Wiley products, visit our web site at www.wiley.com.

ISBN 0-471-42004-2

Printed in the United States of America

10 9 8 7 6 5 4 3

For Bonnie, Will, and Emily
and Madeline, Devin, Sarah, Sean, Chris, Michael,
Amy, and Sue

Those who cannot remember the past are condemned to repeat it.

George Santayana (1863–1952),
The Life of Reason, 1905

In the face of such diseases, the most dangerous experiment of all is to do nothing.

Joseph Stokes Jr., M.D. (1896–1972),
in the *New England Journal of Medicine,* 1967,
in reference to the deaths caused by measles and mumps viruses

Contents

ACKNOWLEDGMENTS

The authors acknowledge the physicians, scientists, mothers, fathers, and friends whose knowledge of vaccines and commitment to children helped to shape this book: Jani Bergan; Shirley Bonnem; Candace Chacona; Christina Chan, M.D.; H. Fred Clark, Ph.D.; David Cobb; Susan Coffin, M.D.; Charles deTaisne, Ph.D.; R. Gordon Douglas, M.D.; Joseph Eiden, M.D., Ph.D.; Ronald Ellis, Ph.D.; Geoffrey Evans, M.D.; Bonnie Fass-Offit, M.D.; Denise Freeman; Richard Gesser, M.D.; Beth Hibbs, R.N., MPH; Maurice Hilleman, Ph.D.; Jacqueline Jenkins; Jennifer Lloyd, M.D.; Kristine Macartney, MBBS; Lois and Phillip Macht; Peggy McGratty; Charlotte Moser; Debrah Goodman Nash; Mindy and Carl Offit; Peter Paradiso, Ph.D.; Larry Pickering, M.D.; Stanley Plotkin, M.D.; Geoffrey Porges, MBBS; Bob Ruffner; Jerald Sadoff, M.D.; Allan Shaw, Ph.D.; Stuart Starr, M.D.; Gina Terracino, M.D.; Judith Thalhcimer, M.D.; Thomas Vernon, M.D.; Barbara Watson, M.D.; Jeffrey Weiser, M.D.; Deborah Wexler, M.D.; Amy Wilen; Susan Wei Winnick; and John Zimmerman.

In addition, we thank Beth Waters, Peter Vigliarolo, Joline Fontaine, Kathy Nebenhaus, Nancy Love, and Elizabeth Zack for their unswerving belief in this project.

Introduction

Almost everyone in this country gets vaccines, and therefore almost everyone has questions about them. People want to know what vaccines are made of, if they work, and whether they are safe. They want to know why there are so many shots and whether they are all really necessary. Mostly, they want to know what they are getting when they get vaccines.

In recent years, new vaccines have become available (pneumococcus, chickenpox); some vaccines have been substituted for others (replacement of polio drops with the polio shot); two vaccines (rotavirus, Lyme) have been discontinued; parents have had fears about the safety of a preservative that was contained in many vaccines (thimerosal); and some literature claimed that vaccines may cause sudden infant death syndrome, chronic joint disease, violent behavior, autism, multiple sclerosis, or diabetes. As a result, questions have been raised.

Recently, a law was passed that requires doctors to explain the risks and benefits of vaccines before getting permission from parents to use them. Unfortunately, doctors, often restricted by a busy schedule, may not have enough time to answer all the parents' questions.

The purpose of this book is to help answer the questions you have about vaccines. We'll explain what vaccines are made of, how they are made, how they work, and the risks associated with them. We'll describe the diseases that vaccines protect against—and why it's still important to protect against them.

We hope this book will help you sort through the misinformation that is occasionally offered by books, newspapers, television programs, the Internet, and well-meaning friends and family. More importantly, we hope that this book will help you make the choices that are best for you and your children.

PART ONE

WHAT ARE VACCINES?

CHAPTER 1

DO WE STILL NEED VACCINES?

Vaccines are medicine's bright and shining stars. Before vaccines, parents in the United States could expect that every year:

- *Polio would paralyze about 15,000 children.*
- *Rubella ("German measles") would cause birth defects and mental retardation in as many as 20,000 newborns.*
- *Measles would infect about 4 million children, killing 3,000.*
- *Diphtheria would be one of the most common causes of death in school-aged children.*
- *A bacterium called Hib would cause meningitis in 15,000 children, leaving many with permanent brain damage.*
- *Pertussis ("whooping cough") would kill 8,000 children, most of whom were less than one year of age.*

Vaccines have changed those horrifying numbers. Now in the United States only about two cases of diphtheria, five cases of birth defects from rubella, and no cases of polio occur annually. Vaccines have prevented more disease and death than any other preventive program in history (with the possible exception of the purification of drinking water).

However, because vaccines have almost eliminated certain infections, some people are reexamining their usefulness. Do we still need vaccines? Do their benefits still outweigh their risks? As you will see in the pages that follow, vaccines should be given for three reasons: (1) Some diseases are so common (pertussis) that a choice not to get vaccine is a choice to risk disease; (2) some diseases continue to infect small numbers of children and adolescents (measles, mumps, German measles, Hib), and a drop in immunization rates would cause new outbreaks of disease; and (3) some diseases have been virtually eliminated from this country (polio, diphtheria), but are still prevalent in many regions of the world and could be imported by travelers or immigrants.

CHAPTER 2

HOW DO VACCINES WORK?

Ed and Emily are both five years old. Emily got a measles vaccine when she was fifteen months old. She had soreness and tenderness for two days where the shot was given. Ed never got the vaccine.

One day, both Ed and Emily were exposed in their classroom to a third child who had measles and was very contagious.

About one week later, Ed became ill with measles. He had a cough, runny nose, and "pink eye." Two days after that, he developed a rash that started on his face and spread to the rest of his body. He had a fever of 104°F and started to have difficulty breathing. His doctor requested a chest X-ray and found that Ed had pneumonia (not at all uncommon with measles). After having to spend about a week in the hospital, Ed, fortunately, got better.

Emily never caught the measles to which she was exposed.

Because Ed caught the measles, he will never get measles again. Because Emily got the measles vaccine, she will never get measles. They are both now immune to measles.

But Ed paid a high price for his immunity. He was very sick for over a week. Emily had only a sore arm.

How did Emily get immunity without first getting sick?

First, we need to understand what happened to Ed and Emily.

What Happened to Ed

Ed caught measles from another child with measles who was coughing. When the child coughed, thousands of tiny droplets were sprayed into the air near Ed's nose and mouth. Inside these droplets were hundreds of measles viruses.

Once the measles viruses entered Ed's body, their mission was clear: to make copies of themselves (or replicate) over and over again. The measles viruses replicated in Ed's skin and lungs, causing Ed's symptoms of rash and pneumonia. By the time the replication process was finished, hundreds of measles viruses had become millions of measles viruses.

While Ed was infected with measles, his body produced antibodies to the virus. Antibodies are proteins that are made by cells of the immune system in the blood and lymph nodes. Antibodies against measles virus helped Ed eliminate measles virus from his body. The cells that made antibodies to measles virus will probably stay in Ed's body for the rest of his life as "memory cells." The next time Ed is exposed to measles, these "memory cells" will make antibodies that will neutralize measles virus before it can make him sick. Because Ed now has "memory cells" specific for measles virus, he is said to be immune to measles.

What Happened to Emily

The measles virus that Emily was given in the vaccine when she was a toddler was very different from the one that Ed caught. Emily was given a measles virus that was weakened so that it couldn't replicate very well. Because it replicated poorly, it didn't make Emily sick.

But the weakened version of measles that Emily was given still caused her to produce antibodies against measles and develop "memory cells" that she will probably have for the rest of her life. When Emily was exposed to the measles virus in her classroom, these "memory cells" made antibodies that killed the virus before it could make her sick. Therefore, because of the vaccine, Emily was also immune to measles.

How Viruses and Bacteria Make You Sick

What happened to Emily is what happens to children when they get a vaccine: they get immunity without getting sick. To know how vaccines do this, we need to understand how viruses and bacteria make you sick.

Viruses and bacteria are like M&M candies.

M&Ms are shells that contain chocolate centers. Viruses and bacteria are shells that contain substances called genes. Genes are simply blueprints that tell viruses and bacteria how to replicate.

One virus can make hundreds of copies of itself in as few as eight to twelve hours, and each newly created virus can do the same. It is easy to see how the hundreds of viruses to which Ed was exposed could become millions of viruses within one week.

Many bacteria make you sick just the way viruses do: by causing damage in places where bacteria are replicating. Some bacteria make you sick by manufacturing a harmful protein called a toxin. In this case it is the toxin, not the bacteria, that does the damage.

Ed and Emily had different experiences because they were exposed to different measles viruses. The measles virus Ed caught from another child (the so-called wild-type virus) formed millions of viruses that caused damage to his skin and lungs. The weakened measles virus Emily was given as a shot (the vaccine virus) formed only hundreds of weaker viruses. Because fewer viruses were formed, Emily didn't get sick. But Emily's body had "seen" enough measles to develop immunity.

To summarize how vaccines work:

- Viruses and bacteria cause disease by replicating inside the body and thus damaging cells such as those in the skin and lungs.

- The viruses and bacteria in vaccines don't replicate well or don't replicate at all.

- Therefore, vaccines don't cause the diseases that are usually caused by viruses and bacteria.

- A child given a vaccine is exposed to just enough of the virus or bacteria to cause immunity (the creation of "memory cells").

- "Memory cells" produce the antibodies needed to destroy viruses and bacteria before they make you sick. These cells often last a lifetime.

CHAPTER 3

HOW ARE VACCINES MADE?

Vaccines are made by taking viruses or bacteria and weakening them so that they can't reproduce themselves (or replicate) very well or so that they can't replicate at all. Children given vaccines are exposed to enough of the virus or bacteria to develop immunity, but not enough to make them sick. There are four ways that viruses and bacteria are weakened to make vaccines:

1. **Change the virus blueprint (or genes) so that the virus replicates poorly.** This is how the measles, mumps, rubella, and varicella vaccines are made.

    The virus blueprint is changed by a technique called cell-culture adaptation (see box on next page). Because viruses can still to some extent make copies of themselves after cell-culture adaptation (and therefore are still alive), they are often referred to as live, attenuated (or weakened) viruses.

"Cell-Culture Adaptation" Is Used to Make Measles Vaccine

Measles viruses normally grow in cells that line the back of a child's throat and in cells lining the lung. The measles vaccine was made by taking measles virus from the throat of an infected child (the "wild-type" virus) and adapting it to growth in specialized cells grown in the laboratory. This process is called cell-culture adaptation. As the virus becomes better and better able to grow in these specialized cells, it becomes less and less able to grow in a child's skin or lungs. When this cell-culture-adapted virus (or vaccine virus) is given to a child, it replicates only a little before it is eliminated from the body.

2. **Destroy the virus blueprint (or genes) so that the virus can't replicate at all.** This is how the "killed" polio vaccine (or polio shot) is made. Vaccine virus is made by treating polio virus with the chemical formaldehyde. This treatment permanently destroys the polio genes so that the virus can no longer replicate.

3. **Use only part of the virus or bacteria.** This is how the pneumococcus, Hib, and hepatitis B vaccines are made. Because the viral or bacterial genes are not present in the vaccine, the viruses or bacteria can't replicate.

4. **Take the toxin that is released from the bacteria, purify it, and kill it so it can't do any harm.** Some bacteria cause disease not by replicating but by manufacturing harmful proteins called toxins. For example, bacteria such as diphtheria, tetanus, and pertussis (whooping cough) all cause disease by producing toxins. To make vaccines against these bacteria, toxins are purified and inactivated with chemicals (such as formaldehyde). Again, because bacterial genes are not part of the vaccine, bacteria can't replicate.

Some Vaccines Are Like Sparring Partners . . .

Most children infected with viruses survive without any problems. These children fought and won the big fight against those infections without being permanently harmed by them. However, not all children are as lucky.

Live, weakened viral vaccines are like sparring partners getting children ready for a fight. Sparring partners engage fighters in a little fight (without hurting them) to prepare them for a big one.

Children immunized with live, weakened viral vaccines (such as measles, mumps, rubella, and chickenpox) are actually infected with a weakened form of the real virus. This weakened form spars with the child and helps cause immunity without harming the child. When it's time for the big fight (meaning when the child is exposed to the natural, or "wild-type" virus), the child is ready and able for the match and wins hands down.

. . . And Others Are Like Vitamin C

Protective immunity against a particular virus or bacteria is often directed against one part of that virus or bacteria. Vaccines that use part of the shell of the virus or bacteria (such as hepatitis B or Hib) or those that use an inactivated toxin (such as pertussis, diphtheria, and tetanus) are examples of immunizations using the critical part of a virus or bacteria.

Many people drink orange juice for the vitamin C or consume the essence of the orange juice by taking vitamin C tablets. This is analogous to vaccine strategies that use the essence of the virus or bacteria necessary for protection. In both cases the purified, final product is made from natural ingredients.

WHY AREN'T ALL VACCINES MADE THE SAME WAY?

Wouldn't it be easier just to use the same strategy to make all vaccines?

Different vaccine strategies are used for different infections. For example, both measles and hepatitis B are viruses. The measles vaccine was made by weakening the virus by cell-culture adaptation. However, it is very difficult to grow hepatitis B virus in cells, so the process of cell-culture adaptation couldn't easily be used to make a hepatitis B virus vaccine. Also, the protective immune response against hepatitis B virus is directed for the most part against just one protein on the surface of the virus (which is not true for measles virus). Therefore, a vaccine for hepatitis B virus was made using just that one hepatitis B virus protein.

HOW VACCINES ARE ACTUALLY MADE (THE STORY OF THE MUMPS VACCINE)

On March 30, 1963, Jeryl Lynn Hilleman, the five-year-old daughter of Maurice Hilleman, said to her father, "Daddy, my neck hurts!" It was one o'clock in the morning. Maurice Hilleman, Ph.D., picked up his daughter, carefully examined her throat and neck, and thought to himself, "Oh my God, she has the mumps." Dr. Hilleman's next move was unusual. He went to his research laboratory, picked up some cotton swabs and several tubes of broth (a nutrient-rich fluid in which viruses are kept alive), and brought them home. He then went back up to Jeryl Lynn's room, woke her up, swabbed the back of her throat, placed the swab in the broth, and went back to his laboratory.

In 1963 mumps was a highly prevalent and highly contagious disease in the United States. Most people knew mumps as a painful swelling of the salivary glands (the parotid glands), which are located just below the ear. However, mumps virus can also cause a number of other serious problems. For example, mumps virus can infect the brain (causing encephalitis) or lining of the brain (causing meningitis) in about half of all children that are infected. As a result, mumps virus was one of the most common causes of deafness in children. Mumps virus can also infect the pancreas, the organ that makes insulin, occasionally resulting in severe diabetes. Dr. Hilleman, at the time the director of Virus and Cell Biology Research at Merck, Sharpe and Dohme Laboratories, desperately wanted to make a vaccine to prevent these serious complications.

Despite Dr. Hilleman's considerable understanding of viruses and how they worked, he needed help to develop the mumps vaccine. This help came from his daughter the night she came down with the mumps. Dr. Hilleman needed to find a strain of mumps virus that *couldn't* infect the lining of the brain or the brain itself, and, fortunately, this was exactly the kind of strain that infected Jeryl Lynn. Now that hundreds of millions of doses of the "Jeryl Lynn" strain of mumps vaccine have been given to children throughout the world, the serious complications of mumps infection have been virtually eliminated from most countries.

How did Dr. Hilleman take the virus that made his daughter sick and create a vaccine to protect other children from this occasionally serious disease?

In the early morning hours of that day in March, Dr. Hilleman took the virus that he had obtained from the back of Jeryl Lynn's throat and inoculated it into hen's eggs. Dr. Hilleman wanted the mumps virus taken from Jeryl Lynn to grow in the cells that were part of the chick embryo. After several days, he removed fluid from the center of the eggs and inoculated this fluid into other hen's eggs. This process was done twelve times. The purpose of growing the virus repeatedly in hen's eggs was to weaken it. As the virus became better and better able to grow in hen's eggs, it became less and less able to grow in children. Dr. Hilleman wanted the virus to grow well enough in children so that they developed immunity, but not so well that they would get sick as a result.

After passing the virus twelve times in hen's eggs (now called level A virus), Dr. Hilleman took some of the virus and grew it five more times in chick embryo cells that were grown in laboratory flasks (level B virus). Next, the level A and B viruses were tested to make sure that there were no other viruses, bacteria, or fungi contaminating the vaccine. The viruses were then tested for safety in experimental animals. When the mumps viruses from levels A and B were shown to be safe in experimental animals and free from other infectious agents, they were approved for further testing in children by the U.S. Bureau of

Biologics. Two years had now elapsed since Dr. Hilleman first isolated the mumps virus from his daughter.

The year was 1965, and it was time to test the mumps viruses from levels A and B in children. To do this, Dr. Hilleman called on his friends and coworkers Dr. Joseph Stokes Jr. and Dr. Robert Weibel, both professors in pediatrics at the University of Pennsylvania School of Medicine and at the Children's Hospital of Philadelphia. Their first challenge was to make sure that the mumps viruses were safe in children. About thirty children per group were injected into the arm with the vaccines from level A or B. Both levels A and B vaccines induced mumps virus–specific antibodies in the blood, but whereas level A vaccine still caused mild swelling and tenderness of the salivary glands in some children, level B vaccine did not. So level B vaccine was determined to be safe. The next step was to find out whether the vaccine would protect children against the mumps.

Dr. Stokes and Dr. Weibel went to civic groups and churches in the Havertown–Springfield area of Philadelphia and recruited about 6,300 children who had never before been exposed to mumps virus. These children were injected with level B vaccine, and the investigators waited for a natural outbreak of mumps virus to occur. The results were dramatic: 97 percent of inoculated children developed antibodies to the vaccine, and 97 percent were protected when an outbreak of mumps swept through their community. The vaccine was licensed by the Federal Regulatory Agency (now the Food and Drug Administration) in December 1967, only four years after Jeryl Lynn Hilleman was infected with mumps. One of the first recipients of the new vaccine was Jeryl Lynn's younger sister, Kirsten.

The mumps vaccine that is administered to children today in combination with vaccines against measles and rubella (see Chapter 10) is virtually identical to the vaccine that was used in 1967.

HARD LESSONS ON THE VACCINE ROAD

All vaccines recommended for routine use in children have a remarkable record of safety and effectiveness. However, the development of successful vaccines is not always as linear and unburdened as that of the mumps vaccine. There have been, on occasion, hard lessons. Two instructive cases are detailed below.

THE CUTTER INCIDENT

Probably the most disastrous event in the history of vaccine making occurred in 1955. The event was chronicled in 1963 in a now classic article in the *American Journal of Hygiene* by Dr. Neal Nathanson and Dr. Alexander Langmuir. The first paragraph of that article is shown below:

> On April 25, 1955, an infant with paralytic poliomyelitis was admitted to Michael Reese Hospital, Chicago, Illinois. The patient had been inoculated in the buttock with Cutter vaccine on April 16, and developed flaccid [complete] paralysis of both legs on April 24. The case was reported by the Chicago Board of Health to the Public Health Service on April 25. On April 26 the California State Health Department reported 5 more cases of paralytic poliomyelitis in Cutter vaccinees. All developed within 4 to 10 days of vaccination and all had paralytic involvement of the inoculated arm. This was the beginning of the Cutter incident.

In mid-1950s America, polio was a common and feared disease. Every year about 15,000 people (most of them children) were paralyzed or killed by this virus. The first vaccine to meet this challenge was that developed by Dr. Jonas Salk. Dr. Salk theorized that if you took polio virus, killed it with formaldehyde, and injected it into the muscles, you could protect children and adults from paralytic polio virus. Dr. Salk's theory was proven correct by Thomas Francis in field trials performed between 1954 and 1955—trials in which about 400,000 children were immunized. On April 12, 1955 (ten years to the day after the death of one of polio's most famous victims, Franklin Delano Roosevelt), the announcement of the success of the polio vaccine made front-page headlines across the country. Six companies were licensed to produce and distribute this "killed," or inactivated, polio vaccine. One of those companies was Cutter Laboratories.

In mid-April 1955, about 400,000 people (most of them first and second graders) were immunized with the polio vaccine made by

Cutter Laboratories. Over the two months that followed, 94 cases of paralysis occurred among those vaccinated, 126 cases among contacts living in the home of those vaccinated, and 140 cases among community contacts. Drs. Nathanson and Langmuir proved that these cases were the result of receiving the Cutter vaccine.

How could this happen? Like the measles vaccine described above, the polio virus used to make polio virus vaccine was grown in cells in the laboratory. In the case of Cutter Laboratories, clumps of these cells had formed and settled at the bottom of the flasks. The formaldehyde that was used to kill the virus was thus unable to penetrate into the center of all the clumps and effectively kill all the polio virus. The result was that live, deadly polio virus was given into the arms of some young children. The fact that there was a problem with the vaccine was made obvious when some vaccinated children developed paralysis in the arm that was inoculated (usually poliovirus causes paralysis in the legs).

The result of this disaster was that more stringent guidelines for the manufacture and testing of polio virus vaccine were put in place by what is now the Food and Drug Administration. Over the forty-five years since the Cutter incident, there has not been one case of paralysis in a child receiving the "killed" vaccine, and the paralysis and death caused by natural polio virus has been eliminated from the United States. The current safety tests required for licensure of polio virus vaccines ensure that the Cutter incident will never happen again.

THE STORY OF THE RSV VACCINE

Respiratory syncytial virus, or RSV, is a virus that infects the lungs of young children, usually those less than two years old. RSV is one of the biggest killers of infants and young children in the United States: 90,000 children are hospitalized and between 4,000 and 5,000 die each year, usually because of severe pneumonia (see Chapter 29 for more details).

Because of the importance of RSV, there has been a great deal of interest in preventing the disease with an effective vaccine. However, early attempts to develop an RSV vaccine were frustrated by some surprising results.

In the mid-1960s, a number of investigators were trying to make a successful RSV vaccine. The most common approach at the time was to take RSV and inactivate it with formaldehyde. The vaccine was given in the muscles of adults and then children to make sure that it was safe. Once the vaccine was found to be safe, infants and young children were immunized to see whether the vaccine protected them against pneumonia caused by RSV.

Every year, outbreaks of RSV sweep across the country, so after the children were immunized the investigators only had to wait for one of these natural outbreaks to occur. What they found took them by surprise. Not only were the children not protected against RSV, but after natural infection, those who were immunized developed more severe pneumonia than those who weren't. Some of those who were immunized and later became infected with RSV had to be admitted to the hospital and artificially ventilated.

The strategy used by these investigators (specifically, to take whole, live RSV and kill it with formaldehyde) had been used prior to 1960 to make successful vaccines against influenza, polio, and rabies, and has since been used to make successful vaccines against hepatitis A virus. The reasons for the failure of the inactivated RSV vaccine remain somewhat unclear.

Because the initial field trials showed that the vaccine didn't work, the RSV vaccine was never licensed or manufactured. It was back to the drawing boards. Although we still don't have an RSV vaccine, recent trials of a new vaccine in children have shown some promise.

CHAPTER 4

ARE VACCINES SAFE?

Whether we realize it or not, we're all gamblers. Risks are present in even the most routine activities:

- *We take a bath, even though every year in the United States about 350 people are killed in bath-related accidents.*

- *We eat breakfast, even though every year about 200 people are killed when food lodges in their windpipe.*

- *We walk outside on a rainy day, even though every year about 100 people are struck and killed by lightning.*

We do these things because we think that the odds are heavily in our favor. We are willing to take small risks to enjoy large benefits. If we wanted, we could avoid many of these risks by simply staying in our home, living in a protective bubble, eating carefully prepared soft foods, and having armed guards at our door. However, with the possible exception of Howard Hughes, few people are willing to do this.

Other risks are easier to lessen. Every day we are at risk of catching viral or bacterial infections. For many types of infections the risks are actually quite high. For example, it is estimated that children less than six years old will have an average of six to eight infections every year. This is where vaccines come in. Vaccines are examples of taking small risks (side effects from the vaccine) to enjoy large benefits (avoidance of permanent disabilities or death caused by infection).

The question about vaccines is, "Do the benefits outweigh the risks?" There is probably no better way to answer this question than to tell the story of the vaccine with the highest rate of side effects, pertussis (better known as whooping cough).

THE PERTUSSIS STORY

The pertussis vaccine was first developed in the mid-1940s. It soon became clear that this vaccine had significant side effects. The side effects from the original pertussis vaccine, the one used in the formulation called DTP (which stands for *D*iphtheria, *T*etanus, *P*ertussis), are shown below:

Mild side effects	*Number of children with side effects per number of doses given*
Pain where the shot was given	1 per 2 doses
Swelling where the shot was given	2 per 5 doses
Fever of 100.4°F or greater	1 per 2 doses
Fretfulness	1 per 2 doses
Drowsiness	1 per 3 doses
Vomiting	1 per 15 doses
Severe side effects	
Persistent, inconsolable crying (for more than three hours)	1 per 100 doses
Fever of 105°F or greater	1 per 330 doses
Seizures	1 per 1,750 doses

Because the risk of side effects with the old pertussis vaccine was high, some parents chose not to vaccinate their children. Was this the right choice? Or, asked another way, were children at greater risk from the vaccine or from the disease? To answer these questions we need only look at what happened to children in Japan in the late 1970s.

In 1975, the Japanese Ministry of Health and Welfare, in response to negative publicity about the pertussis vaccine, imposed a moratorium on its use. In the three years before the moratorium, pertussis caused 400 cases and 10 deaths. In the three years following discontinuation of the vaccine, pertussis caused 13,000 cases and 113 deaths. It should be noted that although the side effects from the original pertussis vaccine were high, no child ever died from pertussis vaccine. The children of Japan proved in a clear and definitive way that the benefits of receiving the vaccine far outweighed the risks.

Today, parents have an easier choice about the pertussis vaccine, because a new one with fewer side effects for infants is now available for use in all children (see Chapter 7).

THE NATIONAL VACCINE INJURY COMPENSATION PROGRAM

Unfortunately, the pertussis vaccine story didn't end with the lessons from Japan. In 1974, physicians working at the Hospital for Sick Children in London reported thirty-six children thought to suffer from a variety of nervous system disorders following receipt of the DTP vaccine. In response to this report, a study was performed in England to determine whether the DTP vaccine caused permanent brain damage. The study was called the National Childhood Encephalopathy Study (encephalopathy means disease of the brain), or NCES. Data from this study were interpreted as showing that the DTP vaccine caused one case of permanent brain damage for every 310,000 doses of DTP given.

The report from England that DTP caused permanent brain damage in children was destructive for two reasons. First, it was wrong. A review of the NCES study by the Institute of Medicine (an independent research organization in the United States chartered by the National Academy of Sciences) showed that the DTP vaccine *didn't* cause permanent brain damage. Second, American lawyers, taking advantage of the fear and misinformation surrounding the vaccine, unleashed a flood of lawsuits claiming that it caused not only permanent brain damage, but also unexplained coma, epilepsy, and sudden infant death syndrome. The burden of defending these lawsuits prompted many vaccine makers to stop manufacturing the pertussis vaccine, and soon there were severe shortages. Because of these shortages, the United States was poised to repeat the mistake made by Japan a decade earlier.

Fortunately, the crisis was averted. In 1986, a collaborative effort among the American Academy of Pediatrics, vaccine makers, parents, and lawyers created the National Childhood Vaccine Injury Act (Public Law 99-660). The cornerstone of this act was the Vaccine Injury Compensation Program (VICP). This program, funded by a federal excise tax on many vaccines, compensated those with vaccine-related injuries and to a large extent protected vaccine makers from lawsuits.

How did the VICP decide what constituted a "vaccine-related injury"? Unfortunately, there wasn't much help from published studies, so the VICP took their best guess. They constructed a Vaccine Injury Table that included side effects that a group made up of scientists, physicians, parents, and lawyers felt were most likely to be associated with vaccines. Compensation by this program was based on a "legal presumption of causation" even if there was no medical evidence showing causation. Based on congressionally mandated reviews by the Institute of Medicine, the table has since been updated to better reflect current scientific understanding of what conditions rarely may be caused by vaccines.

Because of the VICP, the crisis was ended. As a result, vaccine prices stabilized, and vaccine makers in this country not only continued to make existing vaccines but increased expenditures on the research and development of new ones.

"SEEN" AND "UNSEEN" RISKS

We tend to overestimate the "seen" as compared with the "unseen" risks. For example, in 1989, CBS News's television program *60 Minutes* claimed that a pesticide used on apples (with the trade name Alar) could cause cancer in children. This story sparked a panic that resulted in the destruction of millions of dollars' worth of apples and apple products and the loss of farms for many apple growers (even those who didn't use Alar).

Man-made (or synthetic) toxins are a "seen" risk. We know we make them, we know we put them into the environment, and we know where we put them. But the "unseen" risks are actually much greater. For example, there are thousands of natural toxins in the environment. Plants make toxins to protect themselves from molds and plant-eating animals. Some of these toxins clearly cause cancer, and some are highly lethal. Even though trace amounts of these toxins are present in milk, corn, peanuts, and eggs, you almost never hear about them. Our diet contains about 10,000 times more natural toxins than synthetic ones.

The comparison between synthetic and natural toxins can also be made with vaccines and infections. Over the first five years of life, most children will receive many different vaccines. Vaccines are a "seen" risk; we know who makes them, how they are made, and who gets them. But what are the "unseen" risks? Thousands of different kinds of potentially harmful viruses and bacteria are part of our daily environment. Many people would be surprised to know that you are more likely to acquire germs from the money in your pocket than from visiting a friend in the hospital. About half of all paper currency carries infectious organisms.

ARE VACCINES SAFE?

So the answer to the question "Are vaccines safe?" depends on how you define the word *safe*. If you define *safe* as completely free of any possible negative effects, then the answer is no. But nothing is completely safe (not even money).

The better question is, "Do the benefits of vaccines (avoiding infections) outweigh their risks (side effects)?" To answer this question, you need three pieces of information:

1. What are the chances of catching a particular infection?

2. What are the risks of side effects from a particular vaccine?

3. How effective is the vaccine in preventing disease?

As you will see in the sections that follow, the benefits of vaccines clearly outweigh their risks.

CHAPTER 5

WHO RECOMMENDS VACCINES?

Parents are told by doctors that vaccines are "recommended" and by schools that vaccines are "required." Few parents understand how these decisions are made and who makes them.

Three types of endorsement are usually in place before vaccines are given to children: approval, recommendation, and requirement. The agencies and considerations involved in each of these decisions are different.

APPROVAL

Before pharmaceutical companies test a vaccine in children, they must first obtain an Investigational New Drug license, or IND. Approval for this license is granted by the Food and Drug Administration (FDA). An IND license is awarded only if companies have shown that the vaccine is completely safe in animals and is not contaminated with other microorganisms not meant to be part of the vaccine, such as fungi, bacteria, or viruses.

Once an IND license is obtained, the manufacturer tests the vaccine in children to make sure it is safe and effective. This information is then submitted to the FDA for approval (or licensure) of the vaccine. FDA approval is based on two questions: "Is the vaccine *safe?*" and "Is the vaccine *effective?*" Therefore, the FDA is concerned solely with the risk-benefit ratio of the vaccine. Once this approval is obtained, the pharmaceutical company has the right to distribute the vaccine.

RECOMMENDATION

Even after a vaccine has been approved by the FDA, doctors will usually wait until it is recommended before giving it to their patients.

There are primarily three committees that recommend the use of vaccines for children: the Advisory Committee on Immunization Practices, or ACIP (part of the Centers for Disease Control and Prevention); the Infectious Disease Committee of the American Academy of Pediatrics (AAP); and the American Association of Family Physicians (AAFP). Each of these advisory bodies is composed of ten to fifteen physicians and scientists with extensive experience in infectious diseases, immunology, and vaccine research. The data considered by these agencies are broader than that considered by the FDA. Whereas the FDA considers only whether vaccines work and are safe, advisory bodies consider how much vaccines *cost* and how to best *use* them. In other words, whereas the FDA considers only risk-benefit ratios, advisory bodies also consider cost-benefit ratios.

Two stories show how advisory bodies consider the cost and use of vaccines.

The issue of vaccine *cost* is best shown by the varicella ("chickenpox") vaccine. Compared with diseases such as measles, mumps, and rubella, varicella is a relatively benign illness with only occasional serious consequences (see Chapter 12 for more information).

The varicella vaccine was licensed by the FDA in March of 1995. One of the questions that the advisory bodies asked when the vaccine was licensed was, "What is the estimated cost-benefit ratio of the varicella vaccine?" In other words, what is the projected cost of immunizing all children in the United States as compared with what would be saved in health-care costs after immunization? For example, it is estimated that for every dollar spent immunizing children with the measles-mumps-rubella vaccine, about $14 is saved in health-care costs. This is not the case for varicella, where one dollar spent on the vaccine saves about 90 cents in health-care costs. However, if you consider that mothers and fathers miss work taking care of children with varicella, the dollar spent on varicella vaccine saves $2.80 in cost to society. In part because of these societal costs, the varicella vaccine was recommended by the AAP two months after licensure by the FDA.

The issue of vaccine *use* is best shown by the hepatitis B vaccine (see Chapter 11 for more information). The hepatitis B vaccine was approved by the FDA in 1981. The decision by the ACIP at that time was to immunize groups only at high risk of acquiring hepatitis B virus infection, such as health-care workers, intravenous drug users, men who have sex with other men, and people living in the house of someone infected with hepatitis B. By 1991 it was clear that this strategy wasn't working: the number of cases and complications of hepatitis B virus infections in the United States remained unchanged. The reason that the incidents didn't change was that about 30 to 40 percent of people who get infected with hepatitis B are not in high-risk groups! So the ACIP changed its strategy and has now recommended that all infants born in the United States receive the hepatitis B vaccine.

REQUIREMENT

The FDA, AAP, and ACIP do not *require* that vaccines be given to children.

Vaccines are required for school entry by state legislatures, and this requirement is enforced by state departments of health. Unlike the AAP, ACIP, and AAFP, states consider whether it is *practical* to require vaccines for all children within a state. This depends on whether enough vaccine is available for all children within a particular age range, as well as whether enough vaccine is provided at low cost by the federal government to allow immunization of children whose parents can't afford it.

For the most part, all vaccines that are recommended by the ACIP or AAP are required for school entry. However, there are state-to-state differences. For example, although the pertussis vaccine is recommended for use in all infants and young children by the ACIP and AAP, it is not required for school entry in Pennsylvania. The pertussis vaccine is, however, required for school entry in about 90 percent of states in the country. Parents should check with their local school districts to determine which vaccines are required for school entry.

THE RIGHT TO REFUSE VACCINES: PUBLIC HEALTH CONCERNS VERSUS INDIVIDUAL RIGHTS

In the United States there are exemptions to the vaccination requirement. For example, a subchapter of the Commonwealth of Pennsylvania's law requiring immunization for school entry reads as follows: "Children need not be immunized if the parent, guardian, or emancipated child objects in writing to the immunization on religious grounds or on the basis of a strong moral or ethical conviction similar to a religious belief."

The United States is different from many other countries in the recognition of the individual's right to refuse immunizations. There are, however, potential dangers in a country's decision to choose the rights of an individual above the rights of a group. Two examples are shown below.

- Between 1990 and 1991 in the city of Philadelphia, measles infected about 1,600 children and killed nine. Almost all of those cases and deaths occurred in children whose parents belonged to two churches that refused immunization based on religious grounds. The religious group refusing immunization was at the center of the measles epidemic and clearly was linked to the spread of measles to the surrounding community. Members of the religious group made a choice. They decided not to receive vaccines and, therefore, took the risk that their children might suffer severe or fatal infections. Their decision proved tragic not only for themselves, but also for other children in the community. Unfortunately, people in the surrounding community did not have a chance to participate in that decision.

- In 1978 and again in 1992, outbreaks of polio occurred in the Netherlands in members of a Dutch Reformed Church, a fundamentalist group that refused immunization for religious reasons. In the Netherlands the immunization rate against polio was about 97 percent. Not one case of polio occurred in people outside the Dutch Reformed Church. However, not all countries have immunization rates this high. In the United States the immunization rate against polio is about 90 percent, and in some areas of this country it is as low as 35 percent. If an outbreak of polio were to occur in this country in a group that refused polio vaccine, it is not clear that we would be as lucky as the people in the Netherlands.

One could argue that an individual's rights should not include the right to catch and spread contagious and potentially fatal diseases.

PART TWO

VACCINES FOR ALL CHILDREN

CHAPTER 6

WHEN DO CHILDREN GET VACCINES?

Vaccines are usually recommended to be given within a range of ages. For example, the first of three hepatitis B shots can be administered between birth and two months of age. In the schedule suggested on the following page, we have chosen specific ages to give a number of vaccines. There are several advantages to this schedule:

- We recommend that the first hepatitis B vaccine be given at birth. Vaccinating at birth will help protect those children whose mothers are unknowingly infected with hepatitis B virus at the time of delivery (see Chapter 11 for more details).

- We recommend that the MMR vaccine be given at the same time as the varicella vaccine. The MMR and varicella vaccines may be available soon as a single shot.

These recommendations will change as different combination vaccines become available within the next two to three years (see Chapter 28).

A Suggested Schedule for Vaccines			
Birth	*Two months*	*Four months*	*Six months*
Hepatitis B #1	DTaP (diphtheria-tetanus-acellular pertussis) #1	DTaP #2 Polio #2 Hib #2	DTaP #3 Hib #3
	Polio #1	Pneumococcus #2	Pneumococcus #3
	Hib (*Haemophilus influenzae* type b) #1		
	Hepatitis B #2 Pneumococcus #1		
Twelve months	*Fifteen months*	*Eighteen months*	*Four years*
MMR (measles-mumps-rubella) #1	Hib #4 Hepatitis B #3 Pneumococcus #4	Polio #3 DTaP #4	MMR #2
Varicella			
Five years		*Eleven to twelve years*	
DTaP #5 Polio #4		Td (tetanus and diphtheria vaccine)	

CHAPTER 7

DTaP (DIPHTHERIA-TETANUS-ACELLULAR PERTUSSIS) VACCINE

Rachel is two months old. Her mother takes her to the doctor and finds out that there is a new vaccine. The vaccine that used to be called DTP is now called DTaP. This new vaccine, which prevents whooping cough (or pertussis), is now supposedly purer and safer.

Is the new pertussis vaccine safe?

Was the old pertussis vaccine unsafe?

If there really is a question of safety, might it be best if Rachel didn't get any of the pertussis vaccines?

DTaP stands for *D*iphtheria-*T*etanus-*a*cellular *P*ertussis. No vaccine has been more controversial than pertussis ("whooping cough"). This is because the old pertussis vaccine (included in the DTP vaccine) had a high rate of side effects. About 50 percent of children given this vaccine had low-grade fever or pain and soreness where the shot was given. The vaccine was also, albeit rarely, associated with severe side effects such as high fever, seizures, and persistent crying. Although the vaccine was remarkably effective in reducing the number of cases of pertussis, some parents were frightened enough that they hesitated to immunize their children.

Unfortunately, the biggest problem with the old pertussis vaccine was that it was incorrectly linked to other diseases. Newspaper articles and television programs wrongly accused pertussis vaccine of causing unexplained coma, sudden infant death syndrome (SIDS), epilepsy, and permanent brain damage. And some television programs claimed that there were "bad lots" of the DTP vaccine.

Fears of pertussis vaccine have been reduced by a new vaccine that includes a highly purified pertussis component called acellular pertussis. This vaccine was recommended for use in all children in 1997. In this chapter we talk about the differences between the "old" DTP vaccine and the "new" DTaP vaccine and try to dispel some of the myths and fears that surround the pertussis vaccine.

Recommendation by the American Academy of Pediatrics

The DTaP vaccine is recommended to be given as a series of five shots at two months, four months, six months, fifteen to eighteen months, and four to six years of age.

PERTUSSIS

WHAT IS PERTUSSIS?

Pertussis, commonly called whooping cough, is a disease caused by a bacterium (*Bordetella pertussis*). Children with pertussis develop thick, sticky mucus in the windpipe, which causes severe spells of coughing lasting two to three weeks. Sometimes the child coughs five to ten times before breathing in; when the child finally does breathe in there is often a loud gasp or "whooping" sound. Pertussis can also cause severe pneumonia or seizures.

Before the vaccine there were about 200,000 cases of pertussis, causing 8,000 deaths each year in the United States. Now there are about 8,000 reported cases of pertussis, causing about ten deaths each year.

> **Pertussis Is One of the Most Contagious Diseases Known to Man**
>
> Ninety percent of unvaccinated children living with someone with pertussis will get sick. Fifty to 80 percent of unvaccinated children in school with someone with pertussis will get sick.

WHAT IS THE PERTUSSIS VACCINE?

Pertussis is caused by proteins (called toxins) released by the bacteria as well as proteins that are part of the bacteria. Protection against pertussis depends in part on making antibodies to these proteins.

The "old" pertussis vaccine (called "whole-cell" vaccine) was made by taking pertussis bacteria and growing them in broth (a nutrient-rich fluid in which bacteria grow). While growing in the broth, the bacteria would produce toxins. Then both the whole bacteria and the toxins were inactivated with formaldehyde. This whole-cell pertussis vaccine was used in the vaccine called DTP.

There is a big difference between the "new" pertussis vaccine (called acellular pertussis, or aP, vaccine) and the "old" DTP vaccine. The "new" vaccine is made by purifying both the toxins and individual bacterial proteins. The whole bacteria (or whole cell) is not present. That is why this pertussis vaccine is called "acellular." The purified bacterial proteins are then inactivated with a chemical, such as formaldehyde. The new, purer form of the pertussis vaccine is in the formulation called DTaP.

Are the DTP and DTaP vaccines safe?

Until 1997, children were given the DTP vaccine. Now the DTaP vaccine is recommended.

The "old" DTP vaccine had a high rate of mild side effects (see Chapter 4). Most of the side effects were caused by the pertussis part of the vaccine. The DTP vaccine caused pain, swelling, and redness where the shot was given in up to 50 percent of children. In addition, the vaccine commonly caused low-grade fever, fretfulness, drowsiness, and vomiting. The DTaP vaccine was made to reduce this high rate of side effects. With the DTaP vaccine, the rate of these generally mild side effects has decreased from as high as 50 percent to between 1 and 5 percent.

The old DTP vaccine also had some side effects that were more worrisome. The DTP vaccine caused high fevers (0.3 percent), persistent crying (1 percent), and seizures (0.6 percent). These side effects were not permanent. With the new DTaP vaccine, their incidence is dramatically lower.

Unfortunately, the more unpleasant side effects of the "old" DTP vaccine discouraged some parents from giving pertussis vaccine to their children. The DTaP vaccine should relieve those concerns.

Did the "old" DTP vaccine cause epilepsy?

Although this question is easy to answer, understanding it is a little harder.

The "old" DTP vaccine clearly caused seizures. The risk was about one case per 1,750 doses. However, there is no evidence that the DTP vaccine caused epilepsy (a permanent seizure disorder). When children who had a seizure from the vaccine were compared ten years later with children who had not received the vaccine, no difference between groups in the incidence of epilepsy was detected. Similarly, there was no difference in the incidence of epilepsy in children who had received the DTP vaccine as compared with those who had never received it. Therefore, although the DTP vaccine can trigger the first seizure in children who have epilepsy, the vaccine does not cause epilepsy.

The incidence of seizures with the "new" DTaP vaccine is dramatically lower than the "old" DTP vaccine. Several studies have found an incidence of seizures from the DTaP vaccine of 0 percent.

Did the "old" DTP vaccine cause seizures?

For whatever reasons, some children have seizures when they get fever. This disease is called "febrile seizures" and affects about 2 to 4 percent of all children. For these children, any illness that causes fever has the potential to cause seizures. In children with febrile seizures, the fever is usually caused by viruses that cause colds, sore throats, vomiting, or diarrhea. The good news is that febrile seizures don't cause a permanent seizure disorder (epilepsy) and don't cause brain damage. Children usually grow out of having febrile seizures by five or six years of age.

Because vaccines can occasionally cause fever, they can also cause febrile seizures. The "old" DTP vaccine caused high fever (above 104.5°F) in about 0.3 percent of children. Therefore, it is not surprising that it was occasionally associated with febrile seizures. The incidence of fever with the "new" DTaP vaccine is about five to ten times lower than with the "old" DTP. Therefore, the incidence of febrile seizures associated with this vaccine will also be much lower.

Did the "old" DTP vaccine cause sudden infant death syndrome?

SIDS causes thousands of deaths each year in the United States. Because the disease affects children between two and four months of age, a temporal relationship between the receipt of a DTP vaccine and SIDS occasionally occurs. However, several studies that compared children who received the DTP vaccine with those who did not receive it proved that the DTP vaccine did *not* cause SIDS.

Wasn't there a "bad lot" of the DTP vaccine?

Television news shows reported that there were "bad lots" of the DTP vaccine. Reports went as far as showing the lot number of the vaccine. Although these reports generated an understandable amount of anxiety among parents and physicians, there has never been any evidence that such "bad lots" actually existed.

The Food and Drug Administration (FDA) has the authority to withdraw lots of vaccines if there are questions about the vaccines' safety or effectiveness (potency). For example, in 1996–97 the FDA withdrew several lots of the influenza vaccine because of reduced potency. The FDA has never recalled a lot of pertussis vaccine because of problems with the vaccine's safety.

Why can't I just avoid possible problems from the pertussis vaccine by not giving it?

Other countries have at times stopped giving the pertussis vaccine. For example, bad publicity about the vaccine in Japan caused people to stop using it there in 1975.

In the three years before the vaccine was stopped, there were 400 cases of pertussis causing ten deaths. In the three years after it was stopped, there were 13,000 cases of pertussis causing 113 deaths. The frightening consequences of discontinuing the pertussis vaccine caused the Japanese to resume giving it in the early 1980s.

An Example of What Happens When You Stop Using the Pertussis Vaccine		
	Cases of pertussis	*Deaths from pertussis*
Japan 1971–74	400	10
Japan 1976–79	13,000	113

My son was recently in the hospital with whooping cough. At the time our whole family was coughing. Can adults catch whooping cough too?

Pertussis has been shown to be a much more serious problem in adolescents and adults than was previously recognized. Between 900,000 and 1 million adults are infected with pertussis every year. As a result, children usually catch pertussis from adult family members. Unfortunately, adolescents and adults injected with the "old" DTP vaccine had a high rate (about 80 to 90 percent) of soreness, tenderness, redness, and swelling at the site of injection. The "new" DTaP vaccine will probably reduce that problem, and adolescents and adults might soon be routinely immunized against pertussis. Immunity to some vaccines (like pertussis and influenza) fades, so booster doses are important.

PERTUSSIS VACCINE:
SUMMARY AND CONCLUSIONS

THE CHANCE OF CATCHING PERTUSSIS

About 8,000 cases of pertussis causing about ten deaths are reported to the Centers for Disease Control and Prevention each year in the United States.

THE RISK OF SERIOUS SIDE EFFECTS FROM THE PERTUSSIS VACCINE

The "old" pertussis vaccine (included in the vaccine called DTP) had a high rate of mild side effects. Most of the side effects were caused by the pertussis part of the vaccine. The DTP vaccine caused pain, swelling, and redness where the shot was given as well as fretfulness, drowsiness, vomiting, and low-grade fevers in up to 50 percent of children.

The "new" pertussis vaccine (included in the vaccine called DTaP) is much purer and was made to reduce this high rate of side effects. With the "new" DTaP vaccine, the rate of these generally mild side effects has decreased dramatically from about 50 percent to between 1 and 5 percent.

In addition, the DTP vaccine occasionally caused severe side effects, including persistent crying (1 percent), seizures (0.6 percent), and high fever (0.3 percent). None of these side effects were permanent. With the DTaP vaccine, the incidence of these side effects is dramatically lower.

CONCLUSIONS

The "old" pertussis vaccine was rarely a cause of severe side effects, including seizures. The "new" purer pertussis vaccine has significantly reduced and in some instances eliminated these rare side effects.

In any case, the benefits of receiving even the "old" pertussis vaccine clearly outweighed its risks. Because of the negative publicity surrounding the pertussis vaccine, its use was essentially discontinued in both England and Japan in the mid-1970s and early 1980s. Many children died of severe pertussis infection as a direct result of stopping the vaccine. On the other hand, no child has died from the "old" pertussis vaccine.

The use of a "new" pertussis vaccine will only enhance the benefit-to-risk ratio.

DIPHTHERIA

WHAT IS DIPHTHERIA?

Diphtheria is caused by a toxin that is released by a bacterium (*Corynebacterium diphtheriae*). The toxin causes a thick, gray coating at the back of the throat that makes it difficult for a child to breathe or swallow. The bacterium also produces a harmful protein (called toxin) that can invade the heart, kidneys, and nerves. About one out of every ten children with diphtheria infection will die from suffocation, heart failure, or paralysis.

Before the vaccine, as many as 200,000 cases of diphtheria causing 15,000 deaths were reported each year in the United States. Because of the vaccine, only about two cases of diphtheria are reported each year. Between 1980 and 1995, only four children died from diphtheria.

WHAT IS THE DIPHTHERIA VACCINE?

Diphtheria causes disease by making a toxin that is released by the bacteria. Protection against diphtheria depends on making antibodies to this toxin.

The diphtheria vaccine is made by taking the toxin, purifying it, and inactivating it with the chemical formaldehyde. An inactivated toxin is called a toxoid. Toxoids cause immunity without causing disease.

Why should I give my child a vaccine for a disease I've never even heard of?

There was a time when diphtheria was a devastating and feared illness. In 1920 there were 148,000 cases of diphtheria in the United States. In Canada, it was the leading cause of death in school-aged children.

Because of the vaccine, the incidence of diphtheria has decreased from a peak of 148,000 cases to about two cases a year. However, we should not be made complacent by this remarkable success. For example, each year there are outbreaks of diphtheria in eastern Europe, Russia, Brazil, Nigeria, India, Indonesia, and the Philippines. The outbreaks of diphtheria that occurred in eastern Europe and Russia were due to a severe decrease in immunization rates among children in those countries. If we stop giving the diphtheria vaccine in the United States, the disease will be heard from again.

DIPHTHERIA VACCINE: SUMMARY AND CONCLUSIONS

THE CHANCE OF CATCHING DIPHTHERIA

Diphtheria is an extremely rare cause of disease in the United States. Only about two cases are reported each year. Between 1980 and 1995, four children in the United States died from diphtheria.

THE RISK OF SERIOUS SIDE EFFECTS FROM THE DIPHTHERIA VACCINE

The diphtheria vaccine doesn't cause serious side effects.

CONCLUSIONS

The risk of severe disease caused by diphtheria is extremely small, and the risk of serious side effects from the diphtheria vaccine is probably zero.

In addition, when you consider that major outbreaks of severe and fatal diphtheria infections continue to occur in eastern Europe and Russia, and that these outbreaks were due to a decrease in immunization rates among children, it clearly pays to keep children immunized against this rare but deadly infection.

TETANUS

WHAT IS TETANUS?

Tetanus is also a disease caused by a bacterium (*Clostridium tetani*). The tetanus bacteria live in the soil and may enter the skin through a cut or puncture wound. Once under the skin, the bacteria can make a toxin that causes severe and painful spasms of the muscles.

Sometimes tetanus can be fatal. Muscle spasms of the throat can block the windpipe and cause instant death from suffocation. Also, the tetanus toxin can cause severe damage to the heart.

Before the vaccine, about 600 cases of tetanus causing 180 deaths were reported each year in the United States. Now about 70 cases of tetanus causing 15 deaths are reported each year.

A Vaccine for a Disease That Isn't Contagious

The tetanus vaccine is unusual. Tetanus is one of the few vaccines given to prevent a disease that is not contagious. The deadly tetanus bacteria come from the soil and not from another person. Therefore, the risk of infection with tetanus will never be eliminated.

WHAT IS THE TETANUS VACCINE?

Like diphtheria, tetanus causes disease by making a toxin that is released by the bacteria. Protection against tetanus depends on making antibodies to this toxin.

The tetanus vaccine is made by taking the toxin, purifying it, and inactivating it with the chemical formaldehyde.

Can't I avoid tetanus by simply washing cuts very carefully?

Although careful washing of cuts and puncture wounds is important, this does not ensure protection against tetanus. Sometimes it is not possible to reach bacteria under the skin after a deep puncture wound.

Does the series of five DTaP shots protect my children against these diseases for the rest of their lives?

No. Protection from these vaccines often declines over several years. Therefore, the diphtheria and tetanus vaccines should be given about every ten years for the rest of your life. These vaccines (in a preparation called Td) are recommended to be given starting at eleven to twelve years of age. This is the recommended age for adolescents to visit the doctor for vaccines (see Chapter 33 for details).

Vaccines Aren't Just for Kids

The diphtheria and tetanus vaccine (called Td) should be given every ten years beginning at about eleven to twelve years of age.

My fourteen-year-old daughter recently cut herself on a piece of glass while walking barefoot in our backyard. Should she get the tetanus vaccine?

A tetanus vaccine should be given to a child who has a cut likely to be contaminated with tetanus bacteria (for example, puncture wounds contaminated with dirt, soil, or saliva). Children do not need a tetanus vaccine if they have received at least three doses of tetanus vaccine *and* have been immunized within the past five years.

TETANUS VACCINE: SUMMARY AND CONCLUSIONS

THE CHANCE OF CATCHING TETANUS

Every year in the United States, seventy cases of tetanus causing fifteen deaths are reported to the Centers for Disease Control and Prevention. Most of these cases occur in elderly adults.

THE RISK OF SERIOUS SIDE EFFECTS FROM THE TETANUS VACCINE

The tetanus vaccine does not cause serious side effects.

CONCLUSIONS

The tetanus vaccine is safe, and there *is* a small but very real risk of contracting severe or fatal tetanus infection from the environment. Therefore, all children should receive the tetanus vaccine. In addition, because the disease occurs most commonly in the elderly, it is important to get the tetanus vaccine (given with the diphtheria vaccine in a preparation called Td) every ten years starting at about eleven to twelve years of age.

CHAPTER 8

POLIO VACCINE

Andy is two months old. His mother takes him to the doctor and finds out that he is scheduled to receive the polio vaccine. She wonders why it is important for her son to get a vaccine to prevent a disease that no longer occurs in the United States. She also wonders why the polio vaccine is no longer given as drops in the mouth.

In 1998 two different types of polio virus vaccines existed. One was a live, weakened virus that was given as drops in the mouth (the oral polio vaccine, or OPV). The other was a killed virus that was given as a shot (the inactivated polio vaccine, or IPV). For almost forty years, virtually all children were given only OPV. In 1998 that recommendation changed.

The Centers for Disease Control and Prevention (CDC) and the American Academy of Pediatrics (AAP) now recommend that all children should receive IPV.

In this chapter we talk about why the oral polio vaccine is no longer recommended for use in this country, and why it is still important to give the polio vaccine.

Recommendation by the American Academy of Pediatrics and the CDC

The inactivated polio vaccine (IPV) is recommended to be given as a series of four shots at two months, four months, six to eighteen months, and four to six years of age.

WHAT IS POLIO?

Polio is caused by a virus. Most people who become infected with natural (or "wild-type") polio virus never get sick. Others will have a sore throat, cough, fever, stomach pain, vomiting, or a stiff neck and headache.

About one out of every 1,000 people who get natural polio infection will be paralyzed. Usually the legs and arms are paralyzed, but the muscles that assist breathing can become paralyzed, too.

Before the polio vaccine, there were 13,000 to 20,000 people paralyzed and about 1,000 people killed each year in the United States by polio. Most of these victims were elementary school children.

Because of polio vaccine (first given in the United States in 1955), natural polio virus infections have been eliminated from this country.

The Horror of Polio

"During her first night in the hospital, when the virus had raged through her body, deadening muscle after muscle but leaving her body on fire with pain, doctors had performed an emergency tracheotomy to keep her from suffocating. . . .

Her throat muscles useless, she was unable to breathe, cough, or swallow on her own. . . . Mother was among the sickest, highest-risk polio patients."

Kathryn Black, *In the Shadow of Polio,* 1996

WHAT IS THE POLIO VACCINE?

There were two polio virus vaccines: the inactivated polio vaccine (IPV) (given as a shot) and the oral polio vaccine (OPV) (given as a pink liquid by mouth). To know how these two polio vaccines worked, you need to know how polio virus makes children sick.

Polio virus first infects a child after entering the mouth and then grows, or replicates, in the intestines. The virus then leaves the intestines, enters the bloodstream, and sometimes travels to the brain and spinal cord (the nervous system). Once in the nervous system, the virus replicates again, damages the nerves, and causes paralysis. Polio grows in the intestines or in the nervous system according to an internal blueprint (the genes).

IPV is made by killing the virus with the chemical formaldehyde. IPV is given as a shot and causes antibodies to be made in the bloodstream, but not in the intestines. Because natural polio virus travels to the bloodstream only after it replicates in the intestines, IPV creates a second line of defense in the bloodstream against future polio infections.

OPV was made by changing the blueprint so that the virus could still grow in the intestines but couldn't grow in the nervous system. Because OPV was given by mouth, antibodies were made at the intestinal surface as well as in the blood. Because the intestines are the first place that polio virus grows, OPV created a first line of defense in the intestines against future polio infections.

Why were there two polio vaccines?

The first polio vaccine made in this country was IPV. This vaccine, made by Dr. Jonas Salk, was first given in 1955. Because of the Salk vaccine, the number of cases of paralysis from polio decreased from 20,000 in 1952 to about 1,600 in 1960.

The second polio vaccine made was OPV. This vaccine was made by Dr. Albert Sabin and was first given in the United States in 1961.

By 1963 there were two polio vaccines available in the United States. As a result, this country was faced with a decision. Which of these two vaccines should be used?

OPV was chosen for three reasons:

1. OPV worked better than IPV at that time. One hundred percent of children given OPV were protected against natural polio, as compared with about 80 percent given IPV.

2. OPV was better than IPV at stopping the spread of polio.

3. Children immunized with OPV often spread the vaccine virus (and consequently immunity) to other children and adults living in the home (known as "contact immunity").

As it turned out, the decision in 1963 to recommend only OPV was the right one. Epidemics of polio were stopped, and there has not been a case of paralysis from natural polio virus in the United States since 1979.

Were the polio vaccines safe?

IPV was completely safe. A small number of children given this vaccine had pain where the shot was given.

OPV, on the other hand, had an extremely rare but very dangerous side effect. About one in 750,000 children given their first dose of OPV either were paralyzed or spread the altered vaccine virus to someone living in the home or community, who then became paralyzed.

Every year in the United States, the oral polio vaccine caused about four to eight cases of permanent paralysis.

Why did the polio vaccine recommendation change?

In the early 1950s, epidemics of polio occurred every year. In 1955, IPV was introduced in the United States and the incidence of paralysis from polio was reduced by 90 percent; epidemics were virtually halted by the end of the decade. OPV became available in 1961 and until 1998 was the nation's primary polio vaccine.

However, two important things have happened since the 1950s that led to the change in the polio vaccine recommendation. First, the polio virus was eliminated not only from the United States, but also from the Western Hemisphere: there has not been a case of natural polio in the United States since 1979 or in the Americas since 1991. Second, IPV was improved.

The new IPV is called *eIPV*, which stands for enhanced-potency inactivated polio vaccine. The new inactivated vaccine is enhanced in that there is a greater quantity of purified, inactivated polio virus in the preparation. The greater quantity of polio virus induces both greater quantities of virus-specific antibodies and a higher level of protection against polio disease than was seen with the original Salk vaccine.

If we don't see polio anymore in this country, why should I give my child the polio vaccine?

Although polio virus has been eliminated from the Western Hemisphere, it has not been eliminated from the rest of the world. Outbreaks of polio continue to occur in Asia and Africa. Because global travel is more widespread now than ever before, an outbreak of polio in this country could be imported. Indeed, the recent events in Afghanistan have severely slowed efforts to eliminate polio in the region.

The World Health Organization, through extensive worldwide use of OPV in Asia and Africa, has targeted polio virus for elimination.

POLIO VACCINE: SUMMARY AND CONCLUSIONS

THE CHANCE OF CATCHING POLIO

Natural or "wild-type" polio has not occurred in the United States since 1979 or in the Western Hemisphere since 1991. The only real chance of catching polio is through contact with an infected person who traveled recently to a country where polio still occurs.

Therefore, the chance of catching polio in this country approaches zero.

THE RISK OF SERIOUS SIDE EFFECTS FROM THE POLIO VACCINE

The inactivated polio vaccine, or IPV, does not have serious side effects.

Conclusions

Because polio virus continues to paralyze and kill children and adults in Asia and Africa, and because global travel is common, importation of polio virus and its attendant horrors remain a very real threat. Given that IPV does not have any serious side effects, the benefits of IPV clearly outweigh its risks.

CHAPTER 9

HIB VACCINE ("THE MENINGITIS VACCINE")

Jessica is two months old. Her mother is told by the doctor that she will be getting a vaccine called "Hib" that prevents meningitis. Does this mean that Jessica will never catch meningitis?

Hib stands for *Haemophilus influenzae* type b, a bacterium that is a common cause of bacterial meningitis. This vaccine was licensed for use in all children less than five years old in 1990, and the results have been dramatic. Cases of Hib meningitis in the United States have decreased from 15,000 per year to fewer than 200, and deaths from Hib meningitis have decreased from 500 a year to fewer than five.

WHAT IS HIB?

Haemophilus influenzae type b (Hib) infects the lining of the brain, causing meningitis. The infection begins with high fever, decreased appetite, and irritability. The child then becomes drowsy and may get a

Recommendation by the American Academy of Pediatrics

The Hib vaccine is recommended to be given as a series of shots to all children under five years of age.

There are three pharmaceutical companies that make the Hib vaccine used for infants. Two of the vaccines are given as a series of four shots at two, four, six, and twelve to fifteen months of age. One Hib vaccine is given as a series of three shots at two, four, and twelve to fifteen months of age.

stiff neck or a headache. Hib can also cause sepsis (bloodstream infection), with symptoms of fever, low blood pressure, and shock. Usually Hib infects children under two years of age.

Even though we have antibiotics to treat Hib, one out of every twenty children with Hib meningitis will die from the disease. Also, about one out of every five children who survive Hib meningitis will be left blind, deaf, mentally retarded, or learning disabled. Obviously, it makes more sense to prevent Hib meningitis with a vaccine than to treat it with an antibiotic.

Hib can also cause severe swelling of a tissue (the epiglottis) that helps close the windpipe when we swallow. Children with infection of the epiglottis (called epiglottitis) can die from suffocation. In addition, Hib can cause severe infection of the joints (arthritis) and bones (osteomyelitis).

What Is the Hib Vaccine?

The Hib bacterium is coated with a complex sugar called a polysaccharide. To be protected against Hib, you need immunity to this sugar. Unfortunately, infants and children under two years of age can't develop immunity to this sugar. Even children who get Hib meningitis at a young age are not immune after infection. However, researchers found that if you join the sugar to a harmless protein (in a conjugate vaccine), children develop immunity to the sugar and are protected against Hib.

Is Meningitis Contagious?

Yes! Young children exposed to a brother or sister with Hib infection are 500 times more likely to get meningitis than children whose siblings are not infected.

Before the Hib vaccine, there were about 15,000 cases of Hib meningitis, causing 400 to 500 deaths each year in the United States. Hib meningitis was the leading cause of acquired mental retardation in the United States.

The current Hib vaccines in this country were first licensed in 1990, and the incidence of Hib infections has been dramatically reduced. As a measure of the importance of the Hib vaccine, four scientists associated with its development were awarded the Lasker Prize (the highest award given in the United States for biomedical research).

Is the Hib vaccine safe?

Yes. Side effects are mild. After receiving the Hib vaccine, about 10 to 15 percent of children will develop pain or soreness where the shot was given, and about 2 percent of children will have low-grade fever.

The Hib Vaccine Is Remarkable

Immunity after Hib vaccination is better than immunity after Hib infection. Only the Hib, pneumococcal, and tetanus vaccines can make that claim.

Will the Hib vaccine prevent my child from getting meningitis?

Meningitis is also caused by other viruses and bacteria. However, meningitis is much more likely to be deadly or cause permanent brain damage if it is caused by a bacterium than if it is caused by a virus.

Before the vaccine, Hib was the most common cause of bacterial meningitis in children. So the Hib vaccine doesn't prevent all cases of meningitis, but it does prevent the formerly most common cause of severe meningitis.

Since the Hib vaccine became available, the two most common causes of bacterial meningitis are pneumococcus and meningococcus. A vaccine that prevents meningitis caused by the pneumococcus is now available (see Chapter 13).

Will the Hib vaccine prevent my child from getting ear infections or sinusitis?

No. Hib is not a likely cause of either ear infections or sinusitis.

HIB VACCINE:
SUMMARY AND CONCLUSIONS

THE CHANCE OF CATCHING HIB

Because of the Hib vaccine, the chances of catching the Hib bacterium, which causes inflammation of the lining of the brain (meningitis), bloodstream infection (sepsis), or pneumonia, have been dramatically reduced.

THE RISK OF SERIOUS SIDE EFFECTS FROM THE HIB VACCINE

The Hib vaccine does not cause serious side effects.

CONCLUSIONS

The Hib vaccine does not have serious side effects, and there is a small risk of getting a Hib infection from others in the environment. Because infection with Hib is often severe and occasionally fatal, all children should receive the Hib vaccine.

CHAPTER 10

MMR (MEASLES-MUMPS-RUBELLA) VACCINE

Joseph is fifteen years old. Joseph's mother recently found out about an outbreak of measles in his high school.

Joseph got a measles vaccine when he was one year old. Will the vaccine Joseph received fourteen years ago protect him from getting measles at school?

Why are all children these days getting two doses of the measles vaccine instead of one?

MMR stands for *Measles-Mumps-Rubella.*

The combination of measles, mumps, and rubella ("German measles") vaccines has been around for almost thirty years and has had an amazing impact on the health of children.

Because of the MMR vaccine, the incidence of deaths in the United States caused by measles has decreased from 3,000 a year to almost none, of encephalitis (inflammation of the brain) caused by mumps virus from 400 a year to fewer than five, and of birth defects and mental retardation caused by rubella from 20,000 a year to two.

Recommendation by the American Academy of Pediatrics

The MMR vaccine is recommended to be given in the form of two shots. The first shot is given at twelve to fifteen months of age, and the second shot is given at four to six years of age.

MEASLES

WHAT IS MEASLES?

Measles is a disease caused by a virus. It usually begins with a cough, runny nose, fever, and "pink eye." A rash then appears on the face, spreads to the rest of the body, and lasts for about five days. Many children develop severe water loss (or dehydration) from the infection.

A devastating consequence of measles is pneumonia, affecting about 5 percent of young children infected with the virus. In Philadelphia, nine children died of measles between 1990 and 1991; most of them died of pneumonia. None of these children had received the measles vaccine.

In older children, measles can cause an infection of the brain called encephalitis, which can lead to brain damage. Although only about one out of every thousand children infected with measles develops encephalitis, 25 percent of those children will have permanent brain damage.

Before the vaccine, there were about 3 to 4 million cases of measles causing 3,000 deaths each year in the United States. Now there are only about 100 cases of measles each year and almost no reported deaths.

WHAT IS THE MEASLES VACCINE?

The measles virus normally grows in cells that line the back of a child's throat and in cells lining the lungs. The measles vaccine was made by taking measles virus from the throat of an infected child and adapting it to grow in specialized cells grown in the laboratory. The cells in which measles virus vaccine was grown were chick embryo cells. As the virus became better and better able to grow in chick embryo cells, it became less and less able to grow in a child's skin or lungs. When this cell-culture adapted virus (or vaccine virus) was given to children, it replicated only a little before it was eliminated from the body.

Because the measles virus can still replicate a little in the child (meaning the vaccine virus is still alive), it is called a live, weakened (or attenuated) vaccine.

Before and After the Measles Vaccine		
	Before the vaccine (1962)	*After the vaccine (2001)*
Cases of measles	4,000,000	81
Hospitalizations	48,000	0
Deaths	3,000	0

Is the measles vaccine safe?

Hundreds of millions of doses of measles vaccine were administered in the United States since the vaccine was first administered in 1963. The record of safety for this vaccine is excellent.

Fever in excess of 103°F occurs in about 5 to 15 percent of immunized children. The fever usually begins five to twelve days after administration of the vaccine.

Rash develops in about 5 to 10 percent of immunized children and is short-lived. Some parents worry that this rash may mean that their child is contagious. However, the weakened measles virus (vaccine virus) is not detected in the throat, respiratory tract, or skin, and transmission of measles vaccine virus from one person to another has not been documented.

Because the measles virus is grown in chick embryo cells, children with egg allergies were at one time advised not to receive the vaccine.

However, recent studies found that the measles vaccine *can* be given to children with severe egg allergies without serious side effects.

Hypersensitivity reactions (or anaphylaxis) are extremely rare after receipt of the combination MMR vaccine. Anaphylaxis consists of swelling of the mouth, difficulty breathing, low blood pressure, and, rarely, shock. Since reporting of all serious side effects from vaccines was implemented in the United States in 1990 (see Chapter 4), millions of doses of the MMR vaccine have been distributed. Eleven cases of anaphylaxis (and no deaths) occurred immediately after administration of the MMR vaccine.

The measles vaccine can also cause a severe reaction called thrombocytopenia. Thrombocytopenia is a decrease in the number of cells in the bloodstream that are used to help the blood clot (platelets). This side effect is extremely rare (about 1 case per 24,000 children immunized) and is not a cause of death or prolonged hospitalization.

Measles in Colonial America

"That fatal and never to be forgotten year, 1759, when the Lord sent the destroying Angel to pass through this place, and removed many of our friends into eternity in a short space of time; and not a house exempt, not a family spared from the calamity. So dreadful was it, that it made every ear tingle, and every heart bleed; in which time I and my family were exercised with that dreadful disorder, the measles. But blessed by God our lives are spared."

Diary of Ephraim Harris,
Fairfield, New Jersey, 1759

Why do children now have to get two shots of the measles vaccine when they used to get only one?

In 1989, the recommendation from the American Academy of Pediatrics changed from a single dose of measles vaccine at twelve to fifteen months of age to two doses of the vaccine. The second dose is now given at four to six years of age. Ninety-five percent of children are immune after the first dose.

If the measles vaccine induces immunity in 95 percent of people after one dose, why give another? There are three reasons this change was made. First, in the late 1980s only about 70 percent of children actually received the measles vaccine. Therefore, a recommendation for a second dose provided many children with a second chance to receive their first dose of the vaccine. Second, about 5 percent of children who receive the first vaccine won't develop immunity; most of these children do develop immunity after the second dose. Third, children who have an immune response to the first dose of vaccine could get a "booster" effect (a further increase in antibodies) by getting a second dose.

The change in recommendation was an attempt to lower the number of children, adolescents, and young adults who got measles. And it worked. Within ten years of switching from one dose of MMR to two doses, the incidence of measles in the United States dropped from tens of thousands of cases in 1990 to about 80 cases in 2001.

Measles Virus Also Causes a Rare Disease Called SSPE

Subacute sclerosing panencephalitis, or SSPE, is a rare disease of the brain caused by measles virus. The disease begins about seven years after measles infection, when the child develops personality changes, seizures, weakness, brain damage, and coma, leading to death.

Before the measles vaccine, there were about twenty cases of SSPE every year. The measles vaccine has virtually eliminated this disease.

My son was recently accepted to college and told that he had to get the MMR vaccine. Does he really need it?

Measles outbreaks have occurred in high schools and on college campuses. To make sure that young adults are protected at the time that they enter college, the Centers for Disease Control and Prevention has now instructed all states to require proof of either two doses of measles vaccine or evidence for past measles virus infection at the time of college entry.

MEASLES VACCINE: SUMMARY AND CONCLUSIONS

THE CHANCE OF CATCHING MEASLES

Measles cases still occur in the United States every year. As recently as 1990, about 28,000 cases of measles and thirty deaths were reported. Virtually all of these cases occurred in unimmunized people. As an extreme example, in 1990 to 1991, nine unimmunized children in Philadelphia died of measles virus pneumonia.

THE RISK OF SERIOUS SIDE EFFECTS FROM THE MEASLES VACCINE

The serious side effect of the measles vaccine is hypersensitivity (or anaphylaxis). Since 1990, when a system for reporting serious side effects from vaccines was established, eleven cases of anaphylaxis (swelling of the mouth, hives, low blood pressure, or shock) were associated with about 70 million doses of the measles vaccine. So far no one has died of anaphylaxis from the vaccine.

CONCLUSIONS

The chance of having serious or fatal measles disease is extremely low, but the chance of serious side effects or death from the measles vaccine is about zero. Therefore, the immediate benefit of the measles vaccine outweighs the risk. In addition, because measles virus still circulates in the United States, decreased use of the measles vaccine would probably result in a resurgence of measles in this country. Decreased use of the measles vaccine recently in England resulted in outbreaks of measles.

Mumps

What Is Mumps?

Like measles, mumps is a disease caused by a virus. Mumps usually infects children younger than ten years old and begins with swelling of the salivary glands, or parotid glands, that are just below the ear. The swelling usually lasts for about one week.

Mumps also causes an infection of the brain (encephalitis) or of the lining of the brain (meningitis). Before the mumps vaccine, mumps virus was the most common cause of viral meningitis. Because infection of the brain was fairly common, mumps was also one of the most common causes of deafness.

Up to 40 percent of males infected with mumps after the age of puberty develop a painful swelling of the testicles called orchitis. In rare cases, orchitis can lead to both sterility and testicular cancer.

In addition, mumps virus caused an increase in fetal deaths in women infected in the first trimester of pregnancy.

Before the vaccine, there were about 200,000 cases of mumps causing twenty to thirty deaths each year in the United States. Now there are several hundred cases of mumps and no associated deaths each year.

What Is the Mumps Vaccine?

The development of the mumps vaccine is described in detail in Chapter 3.

The mumps vaccine is made in a manner similar to that used to develop the measles vaccine. The mumps virus, which normally grows in cells of the salivary glands or cells that line the back of the throat, is instead grown in chick embryo cells. The virus is weakened when it grows in chicken cells so that it can no longer cause disease in children but can still cause immunity.

Like the measles vaccine, the mumps vaccine is a live, weakened (or attenuated) virus.

Is the mumps vaccine safe?

The mumps vaccine is remarkably safe and is only a rare cause of low-grade fever or pain where the shot was given. Like the measles vaccine, it can be administered safely to children who are allergic to eggs.

MUMPS VACCINE: SUMMARY AND CONCLUSIONS

THE CHANCE OF CATCHING MUMPS

Each year in the United States there are several hundred cases of mumps and no associated deaths; many children infected with mumps will develop a mild infection of the lining of the brain (meningitis) or of the brain itself (encephalitis).

THE RISK OF SERIOUS SIDE EFFECTS FROM THE MUMPS VACCINE

The mumps vaccine does not cause any serious side effects.

CONCLUSIONS

The chance of developing a serious mumps infection is extremely low, and the chance of having a serious reaction from the mumps vaccine is about zero. So the immediate benefit of mumps vaccine outweighs the risk. Also, because the mumps virus still circulates in the United States, decreased use of the vaccine would likely result in a resurgence of the disease. Decreased use of the mumps vaccine recently in England resulted in outbreaks of mumps.

RUBELLA

WHAT IS RUBELLA?

Rubella, better known as German measles, also is a disease caused by a virus. Rubella begins with fever, swollen glands, and a light rash on the face that looks like a mild case of measles. Although usually harmless, the rubella virus occasionally infects the brain, resulting in encephalitis, and causes a decrease in platelets, cells that help the blood to clot.

However, if a woman is infected with rubella virus during pregnancy the results are disastrous. Up to 85 percent of infants whose mothers are infected with rubella in the first three months of gestation will have blindness, deafness, heart defects, or mental retardation.

Between 1964 and 1965 there were about 12 million cases of rubella in the United States, causing birth defects in 20,000 children. Now that we have a vaccine, the number of children with birth defects caused by rubella virus has decreased to about five cases per year.

> ## Girls Are Immunized with Rubella Vaccine to Protect Their Future Children
>
> Rubella vaccine is an example of vaccinating one person to protect another.
>
> We vaccinate girls so that if they become pregnant as adults, their unborn babies will be protected against the harmful effects of rubella virus.
>
> We vaccinate boys to help stop the spread of the virus.

WHAT IS THE RUBELLA VACCINE?

The rubella vaccine is made in a manner similar to both the measles and mumps vaccines. Rubella virus, which normally grows in cells that line the back of the throat, is grown instead in human embryo fibroblast cells (fibroblasts help hold various tissues of the body together). These cells were first obtained from a therapeutic termination of one pregnancy in England in the early 1960s. Embryonic cells continue to grow in the laboratory and are used to make rubella, varicella, and hepatitis A vaccines today. Rubella virus is weakened when it grows in these fibroblast cells so that it can no longer cause disease in children but can still cause immunity.

Like the measles and mumps vaccines, the rubella vaccine is a live, weakened (or attenuated) virus.

The Link Between Rubella Virus and Birth Defects

McAlister Gregg was the first person to realize that rubella virus caused birth defects.

"In the first half of the year, 1941, an unusual number of cases of congenital cataracts made their appearance in Sydney. . . . By a calculation from the date of birth of the baby it was estimated that the early period of pregnancy corresponded with the . . . very widespread and severe epidemic in 1940 of the so-called German measles.

"In each new case it was found that the mother had suffered from that disease early in her pregnancy. . . . In some cases she had not at that time yet realized that she was pregnant."

N. McAlister Gregg,
Australian ophthalmologist, 1941

Is the rubella vaccine safe?

Low-grade fever occurs in about 1 percent of those vaccinated and a mild rash in about 5 percent. Children who have a rash from the rubella vaccine are not contagious and do not need to be isolated from pregnant women.

About 15 percent of adult women who are immunized with rubella vaccine will develop swelling and pain in the joints (arthritis). The arthritis is short-lived, or acute, and usually affects knees and fingers. This is not surprising when you consider that about 70 percent of adult women naturally infected with rubella will develop acute arthritis.

Fortunately, arthritis from the rubella vaccine is extremely rare in children younger than fourteen years of age.

If a woman accidentally gets the rubella vaccine when she is pregnant, can her baby get birth defects?

So far there has never been a child who suffered birth defects because a rubella vaccine was given during pregnancy—and the vaccine has been mistakenly given during more than 1,000 pregnancies. However, because it is theoretically possible that the rubella vaccine could cause birth defects, it should not be given to pregnant women.

Women who plan to conceive usually have their blood checked for the presence of antibodies to rubella as part of routine care. If a woman is not immune to rubella, she should receive the rubella vaccine at least one month prior to conception.

RUBELLA VACCINE: SUMMARY AND CONCLUSIONS

THE CHANCE OF CATCHING RUBELLA

Every year several hundred cases of rubella and about five cases of birth defects caused by rubella infection during pregnancy are reported.

THE RISK OF SERIOUS SIDE EFFECTS FROM THE RUBELLA VACCINE

The most serious side effect from rubella vaccine is the development of short-lived—less than one week, and not chronic—arthritis (or swelling of the joints). This occurs in as many as 15 percent of adult women who receive the vaccine. Fortunately, this complication occurs extremely rarely (probably less than 1 percent of the time) in children younger than fourteen years of age who are given the rubella vaccine.

CONCLUSIONS

Since the introduction of the rubella vaccine, the incidence of birth defects caused by rubella infection during pregnancy has been extremely rare. About two to five children every year in the United States have blindness, deafness, heart defects, or mental retardation as a consequence of maternal rubella infection.

The serious side effect from the rubella vaccine is short-lived swelling of the joints.

Both the chance of serious complications from rubella infection (birth defects) and the chance of serious side effects from the vaccine (swelling of the joints) are very low. But the severity of the consequences of a missed vaccine far outweighs that of receiving the vaccine. In addition, because rubella infections are usually without symptoms, the reported incidence of disease is less than the actual incidence of infection. Decreased use of the vaccine will only increase the chance that pregnant women will be exposed to rubella and that rubella infection could damage their children.

CHAPTER 11

HEPATITIS B VACCINE ("THE HEPATITIS VACCINE")

When William was only twelve hours old, his mother was handed a form by the nurse requesting permission to give him the hepatitis B vaccine.

Wasn't William too young to get a vaccine?

Why was it necessary to give him a vaccine when he was only twelve hours old?

The hepatitis B virus is one of several viruses that cause hepatitis (inflammation of the liver), cirrhosis (severe liver disease), and liver cancer. Every year hundreds of thousands of people in the United States are infected with hepatitis B virus.

Until recently, the hepatitis B vaccine was recommended only for people at highest risk of acquiring hepatitis B virus infection (usually adolescents and young adults). This included health-care workers, intravenous drug users, men who have sex with men, and people living in the house of someone infected with hepatitis B. Unfortunately, this policy didn't work, and the number of hepatitis B virus infections remained unchanged. The policy didn't work because 30 to 40 percent of people who get infected with hepatitis B virus are not in any of these high-risk groups!

In 1991 a new policy was enacted: it was recommended that *all* infants receive the hepatitis B vaccine. Some parents feel that because their children will never be in a group at high risk of getting hepatitis B infection, they should not receive the vaccine. In this chapter we discuss why the policy of immunizing all children makes sense.

Recommendation by the American Academy of Pediatrics

Three doses of the hepatitis B vaccine are recommended for all infants and young children. The first dose should be given between birth and two months of age; the second dose should be given one to two months after the first dose; and the third dose should be given between six months and eighteen months of age.

WHAT IS HEPATITIS B?

Hepatitis B is a virus that infects the liver. Most children infected with hepatitis B virus don't feel sick. A few children have a loss of appetite, tiredness, vomiting, nausea, and yellow eyes and skin (called jaundice).

Hepatitis B virus usually infects adolescents and young adults. Although most people get better, some carry the virus in their bloodstream for decades. These carriers may not look or feel sick, but they can spread the disease to other people. This is why hepatitis B virus infections are called the "silent" epidemic.

WHAT IS THE HEPATITIS B VACCINE?

The hepatitis B virus is coated with hepatitis B surface protein. To be protected against the virus, you need immunity to this protein.

Researchers found a way to purify this protein and use it as a vaccine. Therefore, the hepatitis B vaccine does not contain hepatitis B virus—it contains only a small part of the virus.

The hepatitis B virus is unusual in that when it grows in liver cells, it makes more surface protein than it needs. Blood from infected people contains an excess of this surface protein, and this excess protein can be easily separated away from the infectious virus. In fact, there are about 50 trillion hepatitis B surface protein particles (not attached to infectious virus) in one teaspoon of blood. The first vaccine against hepatitis B took advantage of this phenomenon.

The first hepatitis B vaccine was made by taking blood from people infected with hepatitis B virus, treating it with chemicals that would kill any known infectious agent, and purifying the hepatitis B virus surface protein. The vaccine was used in this country from 1981 to 1992 and was both safe and effective.

Later, to relieve fears that the blood used to make the hepatitis B vaccine might contain other infectious agents (such as the AIDS virus), a different approach was taken. Hepatitis B virus surface protein was manufactured by taking the gene that codes for the protein and inserting it into yeast cells. The hepatitis B virus surface protein made in the yeast cells was separated from them, purified, and used as a vaccine. This genetically engineered or "yeast-derived" vaccine was first introduced in the United States in 1986 and has proven to be both safe and effective. However, because of the way that it is made, the vaccine does contain small amounts of yeast cell proteins.

Is the hepatitis B vaccine safe?

Millions of adults, infants, and children have been immunized with the hepatitis B vaccine. About 3 percent of children develop pain and tenderness where the shot was given; low-grade fevers occur in about 1 percent.

One extremely rare side effect of the hepatitis B vaccine is anaphylaxis (or hypersensitivity reaction). Symptoms of anaphylaxis include swelling of the mouth, breathing difficulties, low blood pressure, and shock. The incidence of anaphylaxis in children is estimated to be about one case per 600,000 doses given. Although it is a serious and frightening side effect, no one has ever died of anaphylaxis from the hepatitis B vaccine.

Because the vaccine is made in yeast cells, those with known allergies to yeast should not receive it.

Will the hepatitis B vaccine prevent my child from getting hepatitis?

Hepatitis is caused by several viruses. However, hepatitis B virus accounts for about 50 percent of all viral causes of hepatitis and is the most common cause of severe liver disease and liver cancer. Most of the other cases of viral hepatitis are caused by hepatitis A virus (for which there is also a vaccine; see Chapter 21).

So, the hepatitis B vaccine does not prevent all cases of hepatitis, but it does prevent the most common cause of severe hepatitis.

Isn't hepatitis usually a mild infection?

Many people infected with hepatitis B never feel sick. However, each year in the United States thousands of people are hospitalized and hundreds die from liver damage caused by the virus.

The "Silent" Epidemic

"The existence of a worldwide pandemic can escape medical detection and public alarm when . . . its natural signs are obscure or separated in time by decades. Such was the case with hepatitis B. Its link to cancer and cirrhosis of the liver, sequelae that take thirty to forty years to appear . . . was entirely hidden. Thus, it was for thousands of years a 'silent' epidemic, whose dimensions and severity went undetected."

William Muraskin,
The War Against Hepatitis B, 1995

In addition, carriers—people who carry hepatitis B virus in their blood for long periods of time—are likely to get severe liver disease (called cirrhosis) or liver cancer. There are currently more than 1 million carriers of hepatitis B virus in the United States. Thousands of carriers die from cirrhosis and liver cancer every year.

How do you catch the hepatitis B virus?

People infected with hepatitis B virus have large quantities of the virus in their blood. In fact, it is estimated that as many as 500 million infectious particles are present in about one teaspoon of blood from an infected person. The most likely way to catch hepatitis B virus is by coming in contact with small amounts of blood from an infected person.

Infants born to mothers who are infected with the hepatitis B virus are at high risk of getting the disease. During delivery, newborns come in contact with large quantities of blood in the birth canal. About 90 percent of newborns infected during delivery will not only be infected, but go on to develop chronic hepatitis B virus infection. Many of those with chronic infection will develop liver failure (cirrhosis) or liver cancer and die from the disease.

Others at risk of catching hepatitis B virus from infected people include intravenous drug users who share needles, health-care workers exposed to blood, and sexual and family contacts of hepatitis B virus carriers. Because blood contains such a high quantity of infectious virus, family contacts are at risk simply by sharing washcloths, toothbrushes, razors, or nail clippers with an infected person. This might, in part, explain why many people who catch hepatitis B virus never know how they caught it.

The Hepatitis B Vaccine Is the Only Vaccine That Can Prevent Cancer

Hepatitis B virus is the second most common cause of cancer (specifically, liver cancer) known to man.

Cigarette smoking is the first.

My son got the hepatitis B vaccine right after he was born. Isn't this too early to get a vaccine?

Newborns whose mothers are infected with hepatitis B virus are exposed to large quantities of maternal blood at birth. Many of these children catch hepatitis B virus, and go on to develop chronic liver disease and die.

Every year in the United States, thousands of women infected with hepatitis B virus give birth. By starting the series of vaccines within the first day of life, most infants born to mothers infected with the virus will be protected against hepatitis B infection.

What is most unusual about the hepatitis B vaccine is that it works even after newborns have been exposed to the virus. If newborns are exposed to maternal blood containing hepatitis B virus during delivery, then the virus may have a twenty-four-hour head start on the vaccine. But the vaccine still works to prevent hepatitis B virus infections in these children. This is because the incubation period (the time from exposure to the virus to development of disease) for hepatitis B virus is fairly long (about seventy days on average).

Are the hep B shots that my daughter gets in her first year enough, or will she need more doses when she gets older?

The new hepatitis B vaccine has been around since 1986. There is no evidence that you need another dose beyond the initial series of three doses.

Why are all children supposed to get the hep B vaccine when only some of them are at risk?

Most people in the United States catch hepatitis B virus infection as adolescents or adults. People catch hepatitis B virus when they (1) have sexual contact with an infected person, (2) take care of an infected person in the hospital (for example, doctors, nurses, medical students, hemodialysis technicians), or (3) live in the home of someone infected with the virus.

Unfortunately, people who transmit the disease often don't know that they are infected with hepatitis B virus and are contagious. It is, therefore, very difficult to know for sure who is likely to get infected. Indeed, about 30 to 40 percent of people who catch hepatitis B virus have no idea where they got it. Every year in the United States thousands of children less than ten years old catch hepatitis B from infected siblings, playmates, or relatives. For this reason, the strategy of selectively immunizing only people at highest risk didn't work in the United States. As a result, the vaccine has been recommended for all children in this country, preferably starting at birth.

My doctor tested my blood at the beginning of my pregnancy and said that I don't have hepatitis B. Why, then, does my baby have to get the hep B vaccine at birth?

Most pregnant women have blood taken to see whether they are infected with hepatitis B in the first trimester of pregnancy. However, hepatitis B virus is a common infection and many people are unaware of how they caught it. So women could become infected during the last two trimesters of pregnancy and pass the infection on to their babies. In addition, infants can catch hepatitis B virus infection from siblings, playmates, relatives, or friends of the family. Many of these people don't know that they are infected. Because infection of infants with hepatitis B virus is often very severe and occasionally fatal, it is recommended that infants receive the vaccine at birth.

My fifteen-year-old daughter did not get the hep B vaccine during her routine shots. Should she get the vaccine now?

The recommendation that all infants born in this country receive the hepatitis B vaccine was made in 1991.

But what about those children who were born before we started to immunize all infants? Aren't they still at risk of getting hepatitis B when they become adolescents and adults? The answer to that question is obviously yes. Therefore, all children who didn't get the hepatitis B vaccine as infants should be immunized.

Hepatitis B Vaccine:
Summary and Conclusions

The Chance of Catching Hepatitis B

Hundreds of thousands of people are infected with hepatitis B virus each year in the United States; thousands are hospitalized and die from liver damage caused by the virus. Although most infections occur in high-risk groups, many people who get infected with hepatitis B virus are not in these groups.

Infants born to mothers who are infected with hepatitis B virus are at great risk of getting infected during delivery and developing chronic hepatitis B virus infection.

The Risk of Serious Side Effects from the Hepatitis B Vaccine

A rare side effect of the hepatitis B vaccine is anaphylaxis, or hypersensitivity reaction. Symptoms of anaphylaxis include swelling of the mouth, breathing difficulties, low blood pressure, and shock. The incidence of anaphylaxis in children is estimated to be about one case per 600,000 doses given. Although a serious and frightening side effect, no one has ever died of anaphylaxis from the hepatitis B vaccine.

Conclusions

The incidence of severe and occasionally fatal hepatitis B virus infection in this country is still quite high. Because about 30 to 40 percent of people infected with hepatitis B are not in high-risk groups, the hepatitis B vaccine is now recommended for routine use in all children.

Every year thousands of people die from hepatitis B virus infection. No one has ever died as a result of hepatitis B vaccination.

The benefits of giving the hepatitis B vaccine clearly outweigh the risks.

CHAPTER 12

VARICELLA VACCINE ("THE CHICKENPOX VACCINE")

Rebecca is one year old. Her mother takes her to the doctor and finds out that a vaccine called the varicella vaccine prevents chickenpox.

The doctor tells Rebecca's mother that chickenpox is usually a mild disease and that she can decide whether Rebecca should be immunized. Rebecca's mother has some friends whose children have gotten the vaccine and some whose children haven't.

Should Rebecca get the chickenpox vaccine?

The varicella ("chickenpox") vaccine was approved for use in children in 1995. Since then it has gradually attained widespread acceptance. It is recommended that some adults receive the vaccine as well (see Chapter 34).

Despite acceptance by most parents and doctors, a number of questions about the varicella vaccine have been raised:

1. Why prevent a disease as mild as chickenpox?

2. If children are immunized, won't the disease occur more frequently in adults?

3. Can the chickenpox vaccine cause shingles?

4. Can adults or other children catch chickenpox from someone given the varicella vaccine?

In this chapter we address each of these questions.

> ## Recommendation by the American Academy of Pediatrics
>
> The varicella vaccine is recommended for all children. The vaccine should be given to children who have not previously had chickenpox as either (1) a single shot between one and twelve years of age or (2) two shots separated by four to eight weeks in children thirteen to eighteen years of age.

WHAT IS CHICKENPOX?

Measles makes you bumpy,
and mumps will make you lumpy,
and chickenpox will make you jump and twitch. . . .

> "Poison Ivy" by The Coasters, 1959

Chickenpox is an infection caused by the varicella virus. The infection usually starts as a rash on the face that spreads to the rest of the body. The rash begins as red bumps that eventually become blisters—a child often will get 300 to 500 blisters during a single infection. The blisters eventually "crust over" and fall off in one to two weeks.

Before the vaccine was made available in 1995, each year there were 3 to 4 million cases of chickenpox in the United States. Most cases occurred in children younger than ten years old.

WHAT IS THE CHICKENPOX VACCINE?

The varicella virus normally grows in cells that line the back of a child's throat and in skin cells. The varicella vaccine was made by taking varicella virus from one of the blisters of an infected child in Japan (the family name of the child was Oka, and the strain of virus in the vaccine is called the Oka strain). The virus was then grown in several different types of specialized cells in the laboratory. The cells in which the varicella virus vaccine was grown included both human and guinea pig fibroblast cells (fibroblasts are cells that help hold tissues together). Human fibroblast cells were first obtained from a therapeutic termination of one pregnancy in England in the early 1960s. Embryonic cells continue to grow in the laboratory and are used to make varicella, rubella, and hepatitis A vaccines today. As the varicella virus became better and better able to grow in these fibroblast cells, it became less and less able to grow in a child's skin or throat. When this cell-culture-adapted virus (the vaccine virus) was given to children, it replicated only a little before it was eliminated from the body.

The varicella vaccine is a live, weakened (or attenuated) virus.

Is the chickenpox vaccine safe?

About 20 percent of children given the varicella vaccine will have pain where the shot was administered. About 10 percent will have low-grade fever.

A rash caused by the varicella vaccine occurs in about 4 percent of vaccinated children. Some will develop a rash where the shot was given, and some will get a generalized rash. On average, when a rash does occur, the number of blisters from the vaccine is about ten.

The varicella vaccine causes a mild rash because it is still a live virus. However, the vaccine virus is so weak that it is not efficiently transferred from someone who got the vaccine to another person. Therefore, the varicella vaccine can be given even to those children who are living in the home of someone whose immune system is weak (for example, family members with leukemia, lymphoma, or other types of cancers). The vaccine can also be given to children whose mother is pregnant.

Why should we prevent a disease as mild as chickenpox?

Although chickenpox is very uncomfortable, most children recover without difficulty. For some children, however, chickenpox can have disastrous consequences. For example, about one out of every thousand children infected with chickenpox will develop severe pneumonia or infection of the brain (encephalitis).

Varicella can also cause birth defects. Birth defects occur in about 2 percent of children born to women infected during their pregnancy and include severe scarring of the skin, shortened limbs, mental retardation, and cataracts.

In addition, varicella has been increasingly associated with skin infections caused by a dangerous bacterium called Group A β-hemolytic streptococcus. This particular bacterium, popularized in the media as the "flesh-eating" bacterium, can cause severe and fatal infections.

Although not often mentioned as a complication of chickenpox infection, many children are left with permanent facial scars caused by varicella blisters.

Before the varicella vaccine, about 10,000 people were hospitalized and 100 died of chickenpox each year in the United States. Most of the hospitalizations and deaths from this infection occurred in previously healthy young children.

Chickenpox Should Not Be a Childhood "Rite of Passage"	
Complications from Chickenpox Each Year Before the Vaccine	
Hospitalizations	10,000
Pneumonia	4,000
Brain infection	600
Deaths	100

A True Story

The mother of a healthy eight-year-old girl took her to the doctor for a physical required for camp. The mother had heard about the chickenpox vaccine and asked her doctor about it. The doctor explained that chickenpox was usually a mild infection and that he didn't feel strongly about the vaccine one way or the other. The mother chose not to give her daughter the vaccine.

Six months later the child developed chickenpox, with a blistering rash and fever. Over the course of several days, she had progressive difficulty breathing and was eventually taken to the Emergency Department. A chest X-ray showed that the child had pneumonia caused by varicella. She was admitted to the hospital.

Over the next two days the girl developed more difficulty breathing and had to be intubated and put on a respirator. A new chest X-ray showed that she had developed a bacterial pneumonia on top of what was already a varicella pneumonia. Fluid taken from the child's lung showed that the bacteria was Group A β-hemolytic streptococci. (These bacteria, popularly referred to as "flesh-eating" bacteria, are occasionally associated with chickenpox.)

The child was in the intensive care unit for two weeks but survived.

My daughter was recently exposed to someone with chickenpox. Could the vaccine still keep her from getting infected?

Recently, the chickenpox vaccine has been shown to prevent chickenpox even after a child has been exposed. If the vaccine is given within five days of exposure, it is likely to prevent or modify chickenpox. So if a susceptible child is exposed to chickenpox, and is at least one year old, the chickenpox vaccine should be given.

My son was given the chickenpox vaccine when he was two years old. Six months later he got a mild case of chickenpox. Does the chickenpox vaccine really work?

Like many vaccines, the chickenpox vaccine is designed to prevent moderate to severe cases of chickenpox. However, about 20 percent of children may get a mild case of chickenpox even after getting the vaccine. Children with mild cases of chickenpox usually have fewer than fifty blisters and no fever. So, the chickenpox vaccine will prevent virtually all children from being hospitalized or killed by chickenpox, but will not prevent all mild infections.

If we immunize children, will they be more likely to get chickenpox as adults?

Like many viral infections, including measles, mumps, and rubella, chickenpox is more severe in adults than in children. Adults with chickenpox are more likely to develop severe pneumonia or encephalitis than are children. As a consequence, adults are fifteen times more likely than children to die from chickenpox. Therefore, it is extremely important to try to prevent adults from getting chickenpox.

Our experience with the measles, mumps, and rubella vaccines has taught us that fading immunity after immunization shouldn't be a problem with the varicella vaccine. After children were immunized with the combination of measles, mumps, and rubella vaccines, the incidence of these diseases decreased dramatically not only in children but also in adults. In addition, the varicella vaccine has been used in children in Japan for several decades without any evidence of fading immunity.

Can the chickenpox vaccine cause shingles?

Shingles is a rash with extremely painful and disfiguring blisters on the face, chest, or abdomen. Hundreds of thousands of cases of shingles occur in the United States each year; most occur in elderly adults.

Shingles occurs only in people who have already had chickenpox. After recovery from chickenpox, varicella virus lives silently in the nervous system. As we age, it becomes more and more likely that the virus will reawaken, or reactivate, and infect the skin.

You can get shingles after either chickenpox infection or varicella vaccine. However, shingles after the vaccine is much less frequent and much less severe than after natural chickenpox.

The Varicella Vaccine Will Probably Prevent Shingles, Too

After chickenpox infection, varicella virus travels from the skin to the nervous system, where it lives silently (or latently) for many years. As we get older, the virus reawakens, or reactivates, and infects the nerves and skin in a condition called shingles. Shingles is incredibly painful and debilitating. Blisters can occur on the face or in the eye and last for several weeks. In addition, shingles is quite common—up to 20 percent of adults will have had it by the time they are eighty years old.

After immunization with varicella vaccine, the virus also probably travels to the nervous system, where it lives latently. But because the vaccine virus is much less likely to cause a rash than the natural (or "wild-type" virus) infection, there is probably less vaccine virus than natural virus traveling to the nervous tissue.

The key question is which of these two viruses you would rather have living in your nervous system: "wild-type" virus, which is well adapted to growth in nervous tissue, or the weakened vaccine virus, which is not.

Evidence gathered over several decades has shown just what you would expect. "Wild-type" varicella virus reactivates more frequently and causes more severe shingles than vaccine virus.

VARICELLA VACCINE: SUMMARY AND CONCLUSIONS

THE CHANCE OF CATCHING CHICKENPOX

The varicella vaccine was licensed in this country in 1995. At the time of licensure, about 3 to 4 million cases of chickenpox infection occurred every year in the United States.

Chickenpox is usually an uncomfortable infection characterized by fever and about 300 to 500 blisters. Most children recover from the infection without problems. However, for some, chickenpox can have disastrous consequences. For example, about one out of every thousand children infected with chickenpox will develop severe pneumonia or infection of the brain (encephalitis).

Chickenpox also causes birth defects in about 2 percent of children born to women infected during their pregnancy. These birth defects include severe scarring of the skin, shortened limbs, mental retardation, and cataracts.

Before the chickenpox vaccine, about 10,000 people were hospitalized and 100 died of chickenpox each year in the United States. Most of these hospitalizations and deaths occurred in previously healthy children. By 2002, seven years after the introduction of the varicella vaccine, a clear reduction in the number of hospitalizations and deaths from chickenpox had occurred. But cases of chickenpox still occur every day in the United States.

THE RISK OF SERIOUS SIDE EFFECTS FROM THE VARICELLA VACCINE

The varicella vaccine has been given to children for over twenty years. The vaccine does not cause serious side effects.

Although it is likely to live silently in the nervous system of vaccinated children, there is no evidence that the vaccine virus is more dangerous than the natural virus. In fact, all evidence to date shows that the vaccine virus is weaker than the natural virus and therefore less likely to cause shingles when the virus awakens, or reactivates.

CONCLUSIONS

Because chickenpox still occurs in the United States, parents choosing not to get the vaccine are risking natural or "wild-type" virus infection for their children. Most children will survive this infection without any problems, but chickenpox is a rare cause of permanent disability and death. In addition, children infected with circulating virus are much more likely to get severe shingles than those who are vaccinated.

The benefits of the varicella vaccine clearly outweigh the risks.

CHAPTER 13

PNEUMOCOCCAL VACCINE

A vaccine to prevent pneumococcal infections was licensed by the Food and Drug Administration (FDA) and recommended for use in all children in 2000. In this chapter we describe pneumococcal infections, the pneumococcal vaccine, and how the vaccine is used.

Pneumococcus is a bacterium that is the most common cause of ear infections, pneumonia, bacterial meningitis (inflammation of the lining of the brain), sinus infections, ear infections, and sepsis (bloodstream infection causing shock) in young children. Before the pneumococcal vaccine was available, thousands of previously healthy children died or were permanently damaged every year by the diseases caused by this bacterium. Pneumococcus causes more bacterial infections in infants and young children than any other bacteria. Worse, pneumococcus is becoming progressively more resistant to the killing effects of antibiotics. Therefore, a safe and effective vaccine for children is of tremendous benefit.

Recommendation by the American Academy of Pediatrics

The pneumococcal vaccine is recommended to be given as a series of four shots given at two months, four months, six months, and twelve to fifteen months of age.

WHAT IS PNEUMOCOCCUS?

Pneumococcus is a bacterium (*Streptococcus pneumoniae*) that is now the most common cause of pneumonia, meningitis, sepsis, ear infections, and sinusitis in children under two years of age.

Before the pneumococcal vaccine, every year in the United States pneumococcus caused about 4 million cases of ear infections, 125,000 cases of pneumonia requiring hospitalization, 2,500 cases of meningitis, and 30,000 cases of bloodstream infection. Most cases of pneumococcal infection occurred in previously healthy children younger than two years old. Every year, thousands of children either died or were left permanently damaged from the diseases caused by this bacterium.

Pneumococcus Is Number One

Until 1990, the bacterium Hib (*Haemophilus influenzae* type b) was the number-one cause of sepsis and meningitis in children younger than two years of age. In 1990, the Hib vaccine was released. Since then, the pneumococcus has become the most common cause of these diseases.

WHAT IS THE PNEUMOCOCCAL VACCINE?

Pneumococcus is very similar to Hib. Both are bacteria coated with a sugar called a polysaccharide. Protection against pneumococcus is caused by antibodies directed against this sugar. Unfortunately, infants and children younger than two years of age can't make antibodies to this sugar.

Researchers found that by joining the sugar to a harmless protein (producing a so-called conjugate vaccine), children developed immunity to the sugar. The Hib vaccine is made by joining the sugar to a protein. The pneumococcus vaccine is also made by combining a protein to a sugar. One of the reasons that it has been hard to make a successful pneumococcal vaccine is that ninety different strains of pneumococcus can cause disease. Fortunately, only seven strains of pneumococcus account for about 80 percent of infections in children. Recently, researchers successfully linked sugars from each of those seven strains to proteins.

The pneumococcus vaccine was tested in about 38,000 infants and young children before licensure. The results were dramatic. The vaccine was about 95 percent effective at eliminating bloodstream infections and meningitis caused by pneumococcus. In addition, the vaccine significantly reduced the number of office visits for ear infections and also significantly reduced the incidence of pneumonia in children.

Antibiotics Didn't Solve the Pneumococcus Problem

In the 1940s, antibiotics were developed and hailed as the final answer to the diseases caused by pneumococcus.

However, by 1960, tens of thousands of people were still dying every year from pneumococcus. Antibiotics didn't always work, because diseases such as sepsis and meningitis are sometimes rapid and overwhelming. In addition, some strains of pneumococcus have become very resistant to antibiotics.

Is the pneumococcal vaccine safe?

Less than 10 percent of pneumococcal vaccine recipients develop redness, tenderness, or swelling at the site of injection.

Does the pneumococcal vaccine prevent ear infections?

Ear infections are caused by several bacteria, one of which is pneumococcus. Studies found that the pneumococcal vaccine caused a 20 percent reduction in severe ear infections (those requiring frequent visits to the doctor or those requiring ear tubes) and a 9 percent reduction in all ear infections.

Some Children Are at Very High Risk of Pneumococcal Disease

Younger children without spleens are thirteen times more likely to get severe pneumococcal infections than other children; for the HIV-infected child, the risk is 100 times greater; and for the preschool-aged child with sickle cell disease the risk is 600 times greater.

PNEUMOCOCCAL VACCINE: SUMMARY AND CONCLUSIONS

THE CHANCE OF CATCHING PNEUMOCOCCUS

The bacterium called pneumococcus is the most common cause of pneumonia, bloodstream infections, ear infections, and sinus infections in children. Although use of the pneumococcal vaccine has caused a decline in pneumococcal infections, every year hundreds of children die or are permanently disabled by pneumococcus. In addition, pneumococcus is becoming progressively resistant to antibiotics.

THE RISK OF SERIOUS SIDE EFFECTS FROM THE PNEUMOCOCCAL VACCINE

The pneumococcal vaccine does not have serious side effects.

CONCLUSIONS

The benefits of the pneumococcal vaccine clearly outweigh its risks.

CHAPTER 14

PRACTICAL TIPS ABOUT VACCINES

FEAR OF SHOTS

Many children are afraid to go to the doctor's office when they know it's time to get shots. However, some techniques can help children through this occasionally frightening experience.

Gina French and her coworkers at the Children's Hospital in Columbus, Ohio, published a study evaluating the capacity of breathing techniques to ease the pain caused by immunizations. Their study was called "Blowing Away Shot Pain." They studied about 150 children between four and seven years of age who were about to be immunized. Half of the children were treated as usual. The other half were told the following: "I know a trick that might make it easier. It is something that children who get lots of shots use. When it is time for the shot you should take a deep breath and blow and blow and blow until I tell you to stop." The child was then asked to practice this technique with the investigator. After the shots were given, the children were asked to evaluate their pain on a scale from "no hurt at all" to "the worst in the world."

Children who had been coached in the breathing techniques rated their pain as significantly less than those who hadn't.

Who Shouldn't Get Vaccines

Any child who has had a severe reaction to a vaccine should not receive another dose of that same vaccine. Severe reactions include difficulty breathing, hives, low blood pressure, or shock and usually occur immediately after receiving the shot.

Also, the live, weakened vaccines should not be given to children with leukemia, lymphoma, other types of cancers, or AIDS. The live, weakened vaccine viruses include measles, mumps, rubella, and varicella.

Vaccinating Children Who Live with Someone with Weakened Immunity

Children living in the home with someone who has weakened immunity (such as leukemia, lymphoma, or other types of cancers) can receive all vaccines that are recommended for children.

Live virus vaccines such as measles, mumps, rubella, and varicella can occasionally be found in the throat of vaccinated children. However, because these vaccine viruses are weakened, and because they are detected in such low amounts, children who are immunized with them are rarely, if ever, contagious. Therefore, children living in a home with someone with weakened immunity can get the measles, mumps, rubella, and varicella vaccines.

Children who receive vaccines that contain only a part of a virus or bacterium (hepatitis B, Hib, DTaP) or a killed virus (IPV) are also not contagious.

Children Who Are Ill

Unfortunately, illness is a common reason for many children to miss vaccines. It is safe to give all of the recommended vaccines to children with minor illnesses. Minor illnesses include low-grade fever, ear infections, cough, runny nose, diarrhea, or vomiting. Several studies found that children with mild illnesses were not at greater risk of side effects and had a similar immune response after immunization as children without minor illnesses.

CHILDREN WITH PREGNANT MOTHERS

Sometimes infants and toddlers are scheduled to receive vaccines at the same time that their mother is pregnant. Children who receive live, weakened virus vaccines (measles, mumps, rubella, or varicella) are not likely to be contagious. Therefore, a child whose mother is pregnant may receive *all* the recommended vaccines.

CHILDREN WHO ARE BREAST-FEEDING

It is unlikely that the antibodies found in breast milk can interfere with the ability of vaccines to induce protective immunity in infants. Therefore, all infants who are breast-feeding may receive all the recommended vaccines.

CHILDREN WHO TAKE STEROIDS

Steroids are occasionally given to children with common diseases such as asthma or poison ivy. Because steroids can weaken the immune system, parents ask whether it is safe to give vaccines at the same time children are getting steroids.

The answer is yes and no. It is safe for children who have received steroid creams or steroid sprays (aerosols) to get vaccines. Vaccines are also safe for children who have received steroids by mouth for less than two weeks. However, children who have received high doses of steroids (meaning more than 2 milligrams per kilogram of body weight [a kilogram is equal to 2.2 pounds] per day of prednisone or its equivalent) by mouth for more than two weeks should *not* receive live, weakened virus vaccines (specifically, measles, mumps, rubella, or varicella). High doses of steroids may decrease a child's ability to fight infection, as well as the ability to build immunity after vaccination.

CHILDREN WITH ANTIBIOTIC ALLERGIES

Some children have severe allergic reactions to antibiotics. These reactions may include hives, difficulty breathing, low blood pressure, or shock.

None of the vaccines contain antibiotics to which children are usually allergic (such as penicillins and cephalosporins). Some vaccines contain trace amounts of antibiotics that are extremely rare causes of allergic reactions and to which most children have never been exposed (specifically, neomycin, polymixin B, and streptomycin).

Therefore, children allergic to penicillin, amoxicillin, cephalosporins, or sulfa drugs may receive all the recommended vaccines.

CHILDREN WITH EGG ALLERGIES

Some children are highly allergic to the proteins in eggs. Allergic reactions include hives, difficulty breathing, and shock.

Both the measles and mumps vaccines are made in cells originally derived from chick eggs. However, not enough chicken proteins are contained in the final vaccine preparation to cause problems. Recent studies have shown that even children with severe egg allergies can receive the measles and mumps vaccines without difficulty.

Children with severe egg allergies should not, however, receive either the influenza or yellow fever vaccines.

PREMATURE BABIES

Most premature infants, including those with low birth weights, can be immunized at the usual chronological age. In other words, a child born two months early should still receive his or her first immunization at two months of age (not at four months of age).

The only exception to this rule is the hepatitis B vaccine. Premature infants (children born within 36 weeks' gestation with a birth weight of less than 4.4 pounds) whose mothers are not infected with the hepatitis B virus should receive the hepatitis B vaccine at two months of age rather than at birth. However, premature infants whose mothers *are* infected with the hepatitis B virus should receive the vaccine at birth, independent of birth weight.

GIVING VACCINES SIMULTANEOUSLY

Because children now receive eleven vaccines routinely, some children could receive as many as four or five vaccines during a single visit to the doctor. This is obviously frightening for children and parents and cumbersome for the doctor. The good news is that several vaccine manufacturers are working on making combination vaccines to reduce the number of shots (see Chapter 28).

All routinely recommended vaccines can be given simultaneously. There is no evidence that giving one vaccine significantly interferes with the immunity caused by another. Nor is there evidence that any of the vaccines increases the rate of side effects of another. Different vaccines should, however, be given at different sites of the body.

MISSED VACCINES

A missed vaccine does not mean that the series must be started all over again. If a dose of DTaP, IPV, Hib, or hepatitis B vaccine is missed, the series of immunizations can be continued after the missing dose(s) is given.

VACCINATING CHILDREN ADOPTED FROM OTHER COUNTRIES

Children vaccinated in other countries should be immunized according to the same schedule as that required for children in the United States. However, a written record of immunization should be provided as evidence that a child has been vaccinated either in this country or elsewhere. The majority of vaccines made in other parts of the world, including developing countries, are produced with adequate quality control standards and are of reliable potency.

CHAPTER 15

COMMON CONCERNS ABOUT VACCINES

It seems that almost every month newspaper articles and television programs depict the horrors of vaccines. The villains of these stories are greedy vaccine manufacturers, disinterested doctors, and burdensome regulatory agencies. The focus of the stories is that children are hurt unnecessarily by vaccines, and the tone is one of intrigue and cover-up.

Perhaps the most dangerous part of these stories (apart from the fact that they may cause many children to miss the vaccines they need) is that the explanations are presented in a manner that seem believable. Below we have listed the most commonly aired stories about vaccines and have tried to separate fact from myth.

CONCERN: Vaccines don't work.

Probably the best example of the impact of vaccines is the vaccine that prevents meningitis caused by the bacterium *Haemophilus influenzae* type b (Hib).

The current Hib vaccine was first introduced in this country in 1990. At that time Hib was the most common cause of bacterial meningitis, accounting for approximately 15,000 cases and 400 to 500 deaths every year. The incidence of cases and deaths per year had been steady for decades. After the current Hib vaccine was introduced, the incidence of Hib meningitis declined to fewer than fifty cases per year! The power of the Hib vaccine is that most pediatricians and family practitioners working today saw its impact.

The story of the Hib vaccine is typical of all widely used vaccines. A dramatic reduction in the incidence of diseases such as measles, mumps, German measles, polio, diphtheria, tetanus, and pertussis occurred within several years of the introduction of vaccines against them.

Vaccines not only work, but they work phenomenally well.

CONCERN: *Vaccines aren't necessary.*

In some ways, vaccines are victims of their own success. Most young parents today have never seen a case of measles, mumps, German measles, polio, diphtheria, tetanus, or whooping cough. As a result, some parents question the continued need for vaccines.

Vaccines should be given for three reasons:

- Some diseases are so prevalent in this country that a decision not to give a vaccine is a decision to risk that disease (for example, pertussis).

- Some diseases are still present in the environment. These diseases continue to occur, but at fairly low levels (for example, measles, mumps, and German measles). If immunization rates drop, outbreaks of these diseases will again occur and children will die from our lack of vigilance. This is exactly what happened in the late 1980s and early 1990s when immunization rates against measles dropped. The result was 11,000 hospitalizations and more than a hundred deaths caused by measles. Now, due to an increase in measles immunization rates, there are only about a hundred cases of measles and no deaths every year in the United States.

- Some diseases have been virtually eliminated from this country (such as polio and diphtheria). However, these diseases continue to cause outbreaks in other areas of the world. Given the high rate of international travel, these diseases could be easily imported by travelers or immigrants.

CONCERN: Vaccines are not safe.

What does the word safe mean?

The first definition of the word safe is "harmless." This definition would imply that any negative consequence of vaccines would make the vaccine unsafe. Using this definition, no vaccine is 100 percent safe. Almost all vaccines can cause pain, redness, or tenderness at the site of injection. And some vaccines cause more severe side effects. For example, the pertussis (or whooping cough) vaccine can be a very rare cause of persistent, inconsolable crying or high fever. Although none of these severe symptoms results in permanent damage, they can be quite frightening to parents.

But, in truth, few things meet the definition of "harmless." Even everyday activities contain hidden dangers. For example, each year in the United States, 350 people are killed in bath- or shower-related accidents, 200 people are killed when food lodges in their windpipe, and 100 people are struck and killed by lightning. However, few of us consider eating solid food, taking a bath, or walking outside on a rainy day as unsafe activities. We just figure that the benefits of the activity clearly outweigh the risks.

The second definition of the word safe is "having been preserved from a real danger." This definition implies that vaccines provide safety. Using this definition, the danger (the disease) must be significantly greater than the means of protecting against the danger (the vaccine). Or, said another way, a vaccine's benefits must clearly and definitively outweigh its risks.

To better understand the definition of the word *safe* when applied to vaccines, let's examine four different vaccines and the diseases they prevent.

Is the hepatitis B vaccine safe?

The hepatitis B vaccine has few side effects. However, one side effect is serious. About one of every 600,000 doses of hepatitis B vaccine is complicated by a severe allergic reaction called anaphylaxis. The symptoms of anaphylaxis are hives, difficulty breathing, and a drop in blood pressure. Although no one has ever died because of the hepatitis B vaccine, the symptoms of anaphylaxis caused by the vaccine can be quite frightening.

On the other hand, every year thousands of people die soon after being infected with hepatitis B virus. In addition, tens of thousands of people every year suffer severe liver damage (called cirrhosis) or liver cancer caused by hepatitis B virus. Children are much more likely to develop these severe and often fatal consequences of hepatitis B virus infection if they get infected when they are very young. For this reason, the hepatitis B vaccine is recommended for newborns.

Some parents wonder whether it is necessary to give the hepatitis B vaccine to newborns. They ask, "How is a baby going to catch hepatitis B?" But before the hepatitis B virus vaccine, every year in the United States thousands of children less than ten years of age caught hepatitis B virus from someone other than their mothers. Some children caught it from another family member, and some children caught it from someone outside the home who came in contact with the baby. About 1 million people in the United States now are infected with hepatitis B virus. However, because hepatitis B virus can cause a silent infection (meaning without obvious symptoms), many people who have hepatitis B virus infection don't even know that they have it! So it can be hard to tell who might be contagious. Worse yet, you can catch hepatitis B virus after casual contact with someone who is infected (for example, sharing hand towels).

Because the benefits of the hepatitis B vaccine clearly and definitively outweigh its risks, the hepatitis B vaccine is safe.

Was the old pertussis vaccine safe?
The old pertussis vaccine had far more risks than the hepatitis B vaccine. The old pertussis vaccine was called the "whole-cell" vaccine and had a high rate of severe side effects. Persistent, inconsolable crying occurred in one of every 100 doses, fever greater than 105°F occurred in one of every 330 doses, and seizures with fever occurred in one of

every 1,750 doses. Due to negative publicity about this vaccine, the use of pertussis vaccine decreased in many areas of the world.

For example, Japan simply stopped using the pertussis vaccine in 1975. In the three years before the vaccine was discontinued, there were 400 cases of pertussis and ten deaths from pertussis. In the three years after the pertussis vaccine was discontinued, there were 13,000 cases of pertussis and 113 deaths! It should be noted that although the side effects of the pertussis vaccine were high, children didn't die from pertussis vaccine. What they did die from was pertussis infection. The Japanese Ministry of Health, realizing how costly their error had been, soon reinstituted the use of pertussis vaccine.

What happened to the children of Japan proved that the benefits of the pertussis vaccine clearly outweighed the risks. Today's new "acellular" pertussis vaccine has a much lower risk of severe side effects than the old "whole-cell" vaccine—therefore, it is even safer.

Was the rotavirus vaccine safe?
The rotavirus vaccine was withdrawn for use because of a problem with safety (see Chapter 26). The vaccine was found to cause a rare but potentially very serious side effect called intussusception. Intussusception occurs when one section of the small intestine folds into another section of the intestine. When this happens, the intestine can become blocked. Intussusception is a medical emergency, and children can die from the disease. The rotavirus vaccine was given to about 1 million children in the United States between 1998 and 1999. About one of every 10,000 children who were given the vaccine got intussusception (a total of about 100 children), and one child died because of the vaccine.

What happened to children who didn't get the rotavirus vaccine? Of the 1 million children who didn't get the vaccine, about 16,000 were hospitalized with water loss (or dehydration) and about five to ten died from dehydration caused by rotavirus. Many more children were hospitalized and killed by rotavirus infection than were hospitalized and killed by the rotavirus vaccine. So the United States had to choose between the risk of the rotavirus vaccine and the risk of natural infection. The Centers for Disease Control and Prevention (CDC) and the American Academy of Pediatrics felt that the risk from rotavirus vaccine was simply too great and preferred to wait for a rotavirus vaccine that was safer.

But let us not fool ourselves into thinking that the decision not to use a rotavirus vaccine rendered children free from risk. Because rotavirus disease is common, the choice not to give the rotavirus vaccine was a choice to allow for continued natural infection with rotavirus. This choice meant that children will continue to be at risk of severe and occasionally fatal rotavirus infection.

Is the pneumococcal vaccine safe?
The pneumococcal vaccine was licensed for use in the United States in the year 2000 and was recommended for use in all children less than five years of age. Some parents chose to take a "wait and see" attitude when the vaccine was first licensed. They reasoned that because the problems with the rotavirus vaccine were not revealed until the vaccine was given to 1 million children, why not wait and see what happens after the pneumococcal vaccine is given to at least 1 million or more children?

However, the choice not to give the pneumococcal vaccine was again not a risk-free choice, because every year in the United States thousands of children get meningitis, bloodstream infections, and pneumonia from pneumococcus. So the choice not to give a pneumococcal vaccine was a choice to risk the severe, often permanent, and occasionally fatal, consequences of pneumococcal infection. Parents should be reassured about the safety of this vaccine because of two facts. First, the pneumococcal vaccine was tested in about 20,000 children before being licensed for use. Second, the *Haemophilus influenzae* type b (Hib) vaccine is made in a manner almost identical to the pneumococcal vaccine, and has been given safely to about 3 million children every year since 1990.

Are systems in place to ensure that vaccines are safe after they are licensed?
The rotavirus vaccine is an example of how rare side effects can be detected. The vaccine was tested in about 11,000 children before it was submitted to the Food and Drug Administration (FDA) for licensure. After the vaccine was licensed and recommended for use, the vaccine was given to about 1 million children.

A system called the Vaccines Adverse Events Reporting System (VAERS) then found about fifteen cases of an intestinal blockage called intussusception soon after administration of the vaccine. This was worrisome enough to the CDC to cause them to temporarily suspend use of the vaccine until it could be determined whether the vaccine did, in fact, cause intussusception. An analysis by the CDC showed that intussusception occurred in about one of every 10,000 children that received the vaccine. Because only 11,000 children had been tested before the vaccine was licensed, it had not been really possible to detect such a rare side effect. The result of the rotavirus vaccine experience is that at least 60,000 children will be tested before the next rotavirus vaccine is licensed.

Several other sources of information about the side effects of vaccines, such as the Vaccine Safety Datalink (VSD), are also available. This database also allows one to determine the "background" rate of side effects, meaning the rate of adverse events in children who don't receive a vaccine. So, in many ways, systems such as the VSD are better than VAERS because they allow one to determine whether a vaccine really did cause a rare side effect.

CONCERN: *Infants are too young to get vaccinated.*

Children are immunized in the first few months of life because several vaccine-preventable diseases infect them when they are very young. For example:

- Pertussis infects about 8,000 children, causing about five to ten deaths every year in the United States. Almost all of the cases are in children *less than one year of age*.

- Children *under two years old* are 500 times more likely to catch Hib meningitis if someone with a Hib infection is living in the home.

- About 90 percent of *newborns* whose mothers are infected with hepatitis B will contract hepatitis and go on to develop chronic liver disease, cirrhosis, and possibly liver cancer.

For these reasons, it is very important for infants to be fully immunized against certain diseases by the time they are six months old.

Fortunately, young infants are surprisingly good at building immunity to viruses and bacteria. About 95 percent of children given DTaP, Hib, and hepatitis B virus vaccines will be fully protected by two years of age.

CONCERN: *It's better to be naturally infected than immunized.*

It is true that "natural" infection almost always causes better immunity than vaccination (only the Hib, pneumococcal, and tetanus vaccines are better at inducing immunity than natural infection). Whereas natural infection causes immunity after just one infection, vaccines usually cause immunity only after several doses are given over a number of years. For example, DTaP, hepatitis B, and IPV are each given at least three times.

However, the difference between vaccination and natural infection is the price paid for immunity (see Chapter 2). The price paid for vaccination is the inconvenience of several shots and the occasional sore arm. The price paid for a single natural infection is usually considerably greater: paralysis from natural polio infection, mental retardation from natural Hib infection, liver failure from natural hepatitis B virus infection, deafness from natural mumps infection, or pneumonia from natural varicella infection are high prices to pay for immunity.

CONCERN: *Children get too many shots.*

Infants and young children commonly encounter and manage many challenges to their immune system at the same time. Twenty years ago, seven vaccines were routinely recommended, and children received five shots by two years of age and as many as two shots at one time. Now that we have eleven routinely recommended vaccines, children could receive as many as twenty shots by two years of age and five shots at a single visit. Many parents are concerned about whether children can handle all these vaccines.

But vaccines are just a small part of what babies encounter every day. Although the mother's womb is free from bacteria and viruses, newborns immediately face a host of different challenges to their immune system. For example, from the minute they are born, thousands of different bacteria start to live on the skin as well as the lining of the nose, throat, and intestines. By quickly making an immune response to these bacteria, babies keep the bacteria from invading their bloodstream and causing serious disease.

In fact, babies are capable of responding to millions of different viruses and bacteria because they have billions of immunologic cells circulating in their bodies. Therefore the vaccines given in the first two years of life are literally a raindrop in the ocean of what infants' immune systems successfully encounter in their environment every day.

It is interesting to note that although children receive more vaccines today than they did a hundred years ago, when only the smallpox vaccine was routinely recommended in infancy, the number of separate immunologic challenges contained in vaccines has actually decreased! The smallpox vaccine contained about 200 viral proteins. If you add up today's eleven routinely recommended vaccines, the number of vaccine proteins and polysaccharides (complex sugars) is less than 130: diphtheria (1), tetanus (1), pertussis (2–5), polio (15), measles (10), mumps (9), rubella (5), Hib (2), varicella (69), conjugate pneumococcus (8), and hepatitis B (1).

CONCERN: Vaccines weaken the immune system.

Natural infection with certain viruses can indeed weaken the immune system. This means that when children are infected with one virus, they can't fight off other viruses or bacteria as easily. This happens most notably during natural infection with either chickenpox or measles. Children infected with chickenpox are susceptible to infection with certain bacterial infections (such as "flesh-eating" bacteria). And children infected with measles are more susceptible to bacterial infections of the bloodstream (sepsis).

But vaccines are different. The viruses in the measles and chickenpox vaccines (the so-called vaccine viruses) are very different from those that cause measles and chickenpox infections (the "wild-type" viruses). The vaccine viruses are themselves so disabled that they cannot weaken the immune system. Vaccinated children are not at greater risk of other infections (meaning infections not prevented by vaccines) than unvaccinated children.

CONCERN: *Vaccines "use up" the immune system.*

Is it possible that all the vaccines given to children in the first few months of life use up the immune system? Certainly, children build immunity to only a limited number of microorganisms (viruses, bacteria, fungi, or parasites). The question is, How many?

Probably the most sensible approach to answering this question was that formulated by Dr. Mel Cohn and Dr. Rodney Langman, immunologists working at the Developmental Biology Laboratory at the Salk Institute in San Diego. They theorized that the number of microorganisms to which a body can respond depends on the number of cells in blood that can make antibodies sufficient to recognize all the relevant parts of the microorganism.

Using their theory, it stood to reason that the number of microorganisms to which one responds depends on one's size. Cohn and Langman estimated that elephants can produce immunity to about a hundred times more microorganisms than humans, and that humans can build immunity to at least a hundred times more microorganisms than hummingbirds. Although this would mean that adult humans could make antibodies to more organisms than infants, the scientists estimated that even young infants could respond to about 100,000 different organisms at one time.

Therefore, the eleven vaccines required for all children will use up only about 0.01 percent of the immunity that is available.

CONCERN: *Some vaccines contain other infectious agents that may damage my child.*

All currently recommended vaccines are tested by pharmaceutical companies under the strict supervision of the FDA. Vaccines are tested for the presence of known viruses, bacteria, fungi, or parasites different from those contained in the vaccine.

When you consider that the 3.5 to 4 million children born every year in the United States receive eleven different vaccines by the time they are six years old, and that some of these vaccines have been in existence for over fifty years, the record of vaccine safety in this country is remarkable.

CONCERN: Vaccines cause autism.

Recently, stories carried by the media have caused some parents to fear that the combination measles-mumps-rubella (MMR) vaccine causes autism. Summarized below are (1) studies used to support the notion that MMR causes autism, (2) studies that disprove the notion that MMR causes autism, and (3) other investigations into the causes of autism.

The "Wakefield" studies

Two studies have been cited by those claiming that the MMR vaccine causes autism. Both studies are critically flawed.

In 1998, Andrew Wakefield and colleagues published a paper in the journal *Lancet*. Wakefield's hypothesis was that the MMR vaccine caused a series of events that include intestinal inflammation, entrance into the bloodstream of proteins harmful to the brain, and consequent development of autism. In support of his hypothesis, Dr. Wakefield described twelve children with developmental delay, of whom eight had autism. All of these children had intestinal complaints and developed autism within one month of receiving MMR.

The Wakefield paper published in 1998 is flawed for two reasons: (1) About 90 percent of children in England received MMR at the time this paper was written. Because MMR is administered at a time when many children are diagnosed with autism, it would be expected that most children with autism would have received an MMR vaccine, and that many would have received the vaccine recently. The observation that some children with autism recently received MMR is, therefore, expected. However, determination of whether MMR causes autism is best made by studying the incidence of autism in *both* vaccinated and unvaccinated children. This wasn't done. (2) Although the authors claim that autism is a consequence of intestinal inflammation, intestinal symptoms were observed *after*, not before, symptoms of autism in all eight cases.

In 2002, Wakefield and coworkers published a second paper examining the relationship between measles virus and autism. The authors tested intestinal biopsy samples for the presence of measles virus from children with and without autism. Of children with autism, 75 of 91 were found to have measles virus in intestinal biopsy tissue as compared with only five of 70 patients who didn't have autism.

On its surface, this is a concerning result. However, the second Wakefield paper is also critically flawed for the following reasons: (1) Measles vaccine virus is live and attenuated. After inoculation, the vaccine virus probably replicates (or reproduces itself) about fifteen to twenty times. It is likely that measles vaccine virus is taken up by specific cells responsible for virus uptake and presentation to the immune system (termed antigen-presenting cells, or APCs). Because all APCs are mobile, and can travel throughout the body (including the intestine), it is plausible that a child immunized with MMR would have measles virus detected in intestinal tissues using a very sensitive assay. To determine whether MMR is associated with autism, one must determine whether the finding is *specific* for children with autism. Therefore, children with or without autism must be identical in two ways. First, children with or without autism must be matched for immunization status (that is, receipt of the MMR vaccine). Second, children must be matched for the length of time between receipt of MMR vaccine and collection of biopsy specimens. Although this information was clearly available to the investigators and critical to their hypothesis, it was omitted from the paper. (2) Because natural measles virus is still circulating in England, it would have been important to determine whether the measles virus detected in these samples was natural measles virus or vaccine virus. Although methods are available to distinguish these two types of virus, the authors did not use them. (3) The method used to detect measles virus in these studies was very sensitive. Laboratories that work with natural measles virus (such as the lab where these studies were performed) are at high risk of getting results that are incorrectly positive. No mention is made in the paper as to how this problem was avoided. (4) As is true for all laboratory studies, the person who is performing the test should not know whether the sample is obtained from a case with autism or without autism (blinding). No statements were made in the methods section to assure that blinding occurred.

Studies showing that MMR vaccine does not cause autism
Four studies have been performed that disprove the notion that MMR causes autism.

In 1999, Brent Taylor and coworkers examined the relationship between receipt of MMR and development of autism in a well-controlled study. Taylor examined the records of 498 children with autism or autism-like disorder. Cases were identified by registers from the North Thames region of England before and after the MMR vaccine was introduced into the United Kingdom in 1988. Taylor then examined the incidence and age at diagnosis of autism in vaccinated and unvaccinated children. He found that (1) the percentage of children vaccinated was the same in children with autism as in other children in the North Thames region; (2) no difference in the age of diagnosis of autism was found in vaccinated and unvaccinated children; and (3) the onset of symptoms of autism did not occur within two, four, or six months of receiving the MMR vaccine.

Subsequent studies by Nathalie Smith published in the *Journal of the American Medical Association* and by Hershel Jick in the *British Medical Journal* found that the increase in the number of children reported to have autism was not associated with an increase in the use of the MMR vaccine.

The largest study to examine the relationship between the MMR vaccine and autism was reported in the *New England Journal of Medicine* in November 2002. About 537,000 children in Denmark who either did or did not receive the MMR vaccine were examined for about six years. The incidence of autism was the same in children who did or did not receive the MMR vaccine.

Studies on the causes of autism
One of the best ways to determine whether a particular disease or syndrome is genetic is to examine the incidence in identical and fraternal twins. Using a strict definition of autism, when one twin has autism, approximately 60 percent of identical and 0 percent of fraternal twins have autism. Using a broader definition of autism (that is, autistic spectrum disorder), approximately 92 percent of identical and 10 percent of fraternal twins have autism. Therefore, autism clearly has a genetic basis.

Clues to the causes of autism can be found in studies examining when the symptoms of autism are first evident. Perhaps the best data examining when symptoms of autism are first evident are the "home-movie studies." These studies took advantage of the fact that many parents take movies of their children during their first birthday (before they have received the MMR vaccine). Home movies of children who were eventually diagnosed with autism and those who were not diagnosed with autism were coded and shown to developmental specialists. Investigators were, with a very high degree of accuracy, able to separate autistic from nonautistic children at one year of age. These studies found that subtle symptoms of autism were present earlier than some parents had suspected, and that receipt of the MMR vaccine did not precede the first symptoms of autism.

Other investigators extended the home-movie studies of one-year-old children to include videotapes of children taken at two to three months of age. Using a sophisticated movement analysis, videos from children eventually diagnosed with autism or not diagnosed with autism were coded and evaluated for their capacity to predict autism. Children who were eventually diagnosed with autism were predicted from movies taken in early infancy. This study supported the hypothesis that very subtle symptoms of autism are present in early infancy and argues strongly against vaccines as a cause of autism.

Toxic or viral insults to the fetus that cause autism, as well as certain central nervous system disorders associated with autism, support the notion that autism is likely to occur in the womb.

For example, children exposed to thalidomide during the first or early second trimester were found to have an increased incidence of autism. However, autism occurred in children with ear but not arm or leg abnormalities. Because arms and legs develop after 24 weeks' gestation, the risk period for autism following receipt of thalidomide must be before 24 weeks' gestation. In support of this finding, Rodier and colleagues found evidence for structural abnormalities of the nervous system in children with autism. These abnormalities could have occurred only during development of the nervous system in the womb.

Similarly, children with congenital rubella syndrome are at increased risk for development of autism. Risk is associated with exposure to rubella before birth but not after birth.

Conclusions

Studies of (1) the genetics of autism, (2) the timing of the first symptoms of autism (home-movie studies), (3) the relationship between autism and the receipt of the MMR vaccine, (4) the nervous system of children with autism, and (5) thalidomide and natural rubella infection all support the fact that autism occurs during development of the nervous system early in the womb.

Unfortunately for parents who will someday bear children diagnosed with autism, the controversy surrounding vaccines has diverted attention and resources away from a number of promising leads.

CONCERN: A mercury-containing preservative (thimerosal) contained in many vaccines harms children.

On October 1, 2001, the Institute of Medicine (IOM) issued a report on the use of thimerosal in vaccines. The IOM advises the federal government on health matters and was established in 1970 by the National Academy of Sciences. The IOM recommended the use of thimerosal-free DTaP, Hib, and hepatitis B vaccines in the United States.

What is thimerosal?

Thimerosal is a preservative that is used in vaccines. It is made of thiosalicylic acid and mercury. The mercury contained in thimerosal is an organic form called ethylmercury.

Why do vaccines contain the preservative thimerosal?

Preservatives such as thimerosal prevent vaccines from becoming contaminated with bacteria or fungi. Preservatives are especially important when the vial of vaccine contains more than one dose (multidose vials). Studies from about fifty years ago showed that multidose vials of vaccines could become contaminated with bacteria. Bacteria in the vial could then be injected inadvertently into the child and cause serious and occasionally fatal infections.

Is mercury harmful?

Yes. Mercury at high levels can damage the nervous system and kidneys. Studies in places such as the Faroe Islands, the Seychelles, and Iraq found that the unborn fetus might be harmed when pregnant women ingest large quantities of mercury contained in contaminated fish or fumigated (disinfected) grain. The form of mercury that contaminates the environment is called methylmercury (not the ethylmercury contained in vaccines).

Does thimerosal contain an amount of mercury that could harm children?

The FDA was recently required to compile a list of drugs and foods that contained mercury (the FDA Modernization Act of 1997). Because some vaccines contain thimerosal, they were included in the list generated by the FDA. The amount of mercury contained in vaccines was then compared with acceptable levels of mercury published by the FDA, Environmental Protection Agency (EPA), Agency for Toxic Substance and Disease Registry (ATSDR), and World Health Organization (WHO).

Cumulative levels of mercury contained in multiple vaccines were not greater than those considered to be safe by the FDA, WHO, or ATSDR. However, the levels of mercury contained in multiple vaccines did slightly exceed those considered to be safe by the EPA.

How did the EPA determine what levels of mercury were safe for children?

The EPA looked closely at a study performed in Iraq where pregnant women were exposed to large quantities of methylmercury that had been used to fumigate grain. The EPA then estimated the lowest dose of mercury that was found to cause neurodevelopmental delay in the fetus whose mother ingested this seed grain. From this they calculated the lowest dose of methylmercury that could possibly harm an unborn child. They then divided this dose by a safety factor of ten to determine the lowest acceptable dose of mercury.

There are many problems with using the study in Iraq to determine levels of thimerosal in vaccines that would be safe in children. First, thimerosal doesn't contain the form of mercury that contaminates the environment. Environmental mercury is usually methylmercury, whereas the mercury contained in vaccines is in the form of ethylmercury. Ethylmercury is excreted in the urine more quickly than methylmercury and is less likely to accumulate in the body. Second, vaccines are administered to children after, not before, they are born.

The nervous system of a child is still developing early in a woman's pregnancy, but by the time a child gets a vaccine, the nervous system is more mature and, therefore, much less likely to be susceptible to the harmful effects of mercury. Third, by including a safety factor of ten, the EPA estimate was very conservative.

Has thimerosal contained in vaccines ever been shown to harm children?
No. Studies have never shown that mercury at the level contained in vaccines causes neurological problems.

If thimerosal has never been found to harm children, why are vaccine makers now making vaccines that don't use thimerosal as a preservative?
Thimerosal is being taken out of vaccines for two reasons. First, single-dose vials have largely replaced multidose vials in the United States. Therefore, the risk of contamination with bacteria or fungi is much lower. Second, other preservatives that don't contain any mercury can be used in some vaccines.

So the main reason that thimerosal is being taken out of vaccines is that it can be. Thimerosal (as a preservative) is absent from all vaccines routinely given to children in the United States.

CONCERN: The hepatitis B vaccine causes sudden infant death syndrome (SIDS).

The ABC television program *20/20* aired a story claiming that the hepatitis B vaccine caused SIDS. They showed the picture of a one-month-old girl who had died of SIDS only sixteen hours after receiving her second dose of hepatitis B vaccine. To the reporters of this story, this proved that the hepatitis B vaccine caused SIDS. Although anecdotes can be quite powerful, they can also be misleading.

Every year in the United States thousands of infants die of SIDS. The hepatitis B vaccine is now routinely recommended for infants as a series of three shots. Therefore, some infants who get the hepatitis B vaccine will invariably die from SIDS—and some will die from SIDS soon after the vaccine is given. But does this mean that children who get the vaccine are more likely to die from SIDS than children who don't get the vaccine?

To really understand whether a vaccine causes problems you need more information. You need to know the incidence of SIDS in those who got the vaccine and the incidence of SIDS in those who didn't get the vaccine. Anecdotes do not provide this information. When the incidence of SIDS is examined in immunized and unimmunized infants, there is no evidence that the hepatitis B vaccine causes SIDS.

Indeed, the incidence of SIDS has decreased dramatically since the hepatitis B vaccine was first recommended for all infants. The reason for the decline is that the American Academy of Pediatrics recommended the "Back to Sleep" program for all infants. Parents were asked to let infants sleep on their backs instead of face down. The result was a dramatic decline in SIDS and proved that SIDS was not related to vaccines.

CONCERN: *Pharmaceutical companies occasionally manufacture lots of vaccines that cause high rates of adverse events ("hot lots").*

Individual lots of vaccines that have unusually high rates of side effects have never been identified in this country. Therefore, specific lots of vaccines have never been withdrawn from use as a "hot lot."

CONCERN: *Vaccine-preventable diseases occur more often in vaccinated people than in unvaccinated people.*

On its face, this statement is actually true. However, it is important to understand why it is true.

Let's take the situation of 100 young adults living in a college dormitory and say that 95 were vaccinated against measles and five were not vaccinated. An outbreak of measles strikes the college campus. In the dormitory, six of the 95 people who were vaccinated get measles, and four of the five unvaccinated people get measles. This would mean that vaccinated people get measles more commonly than unvaccinated people (in this case, by a margin of 6 to 4). However, the risk for measles in the unvaccinated group was 80 percent (4 of 5), whereas the risk for measles in the vaccinated group was only about 6 percent (6 of 95). So, people were much less likely to get measles if they had received the measles vaccine.

Indeed, a study recently reported in the *Journal of the American Medical Association* found that unvaccinated people were thirty-five times more likely to get measles than vaccinated people.

CONCERN: The hepatitis B vaccine causes arthritis, multiple sclerosis, and long-term (chronic) neurologic disorders.

A segment of the ABC television show *20/20* told of children and adults who developed arthritis, multiple sclerosis, or neurologic disabilities following receipt of the hepatitis B vaccine. However, if one event precedes another, it does not necessarily cause the other.

For example, multiple sclerosis commonly has its onset in adolescence and early adulthood. Therefore, if the hepatitis B vaccine is given to adolescents and young adults, some will develop multiple sclerosis following receipt of the vaccine. For some, onset of multiple sclerosis could follow soon after receipt of the vaccine and appear to be related. But the only way to determine whether the hepatitis B vaccine caused multiple sclerosis would be to determine the incidence of multiple sclerosis in those who had received the vaccine and the incidence in those who hadn't received the vaccine.

Several studies have been performed to answer this question, and all have reached the same conclusion: the incidence of multiple sclerosis was the same in those who received the hepatitis B vaccine and those who hadn't.

So, why is the hepatitis B vaccine blamed for all of these problems? When children or adults suffer, we search desperately for a cause. If we can find a clear, discrete cause, then at least we can help other people avoid what we have suffered. No clear cause for multiple sclerosis, autism, violent behavior, sudden infant death syndrome, hyperactivity, Alzheimer's disease, and many cancers has been found. It's frustrating. And vaccines are an easy target. But venting our frustrations by blaming vaccines, in the absence of any clear evidence that vaccines are the problem, will only endanger our children.

CONCERN: Vaccines cause diabetes.

One researcher claimed that infants immunized with a single dose of the Hib vaccine at fourteen months of age were less likely to get diabetes than if they received four doses of the Hib vaccine at three, four, six, and fourteen months of age. He concluded that the risk of diabetes could be reduced if children did not receive vaccines at a young age. Some parents have seen this information and chosen to wait until their children are two years of age to have them immunized. This is unfortunate, because some vaccine-preventable diseases, such as Hib, pneumococcus, and pertussis, occur commonly in the first two years of life.

A careful review of the data, however, found that the analytic methods used in that study were incorrect. In addition, a ten-year follow-up study showed that the incidence of diabetes was the same in those who had been immunized early as in those who had been immunized later. Further, a recent study by the CDC found that the incidence of diabetes was the same in vaccinated as in unvaccinated children. So, no evidence exists to support the notion that vaccines should be delayed.

CONCERN: The DTP vaccine causes a disease that looks like "shaken baby" syndrome.

Small children who are shaken forcefully in rage can develop bleeding around the brain (subdural hematomas) and bleeding on the back of the eye (retinal hemorrhages). Some lawyers have chosen to defend people accused of abusing children by saying that bleeding was caused by the pertussis component of the DTP vaccine. However, no evidence exists to support this contention. Neither pertussis nor the pertussis vaccine cause bleeding around the brain or on the back of the eye—only forceful shaking does this.

CONCERN: The polio vaccine is the cause of AIDS.

Tom Curtis wrote an article in *Rolling Stone* magazine claiming that the origin of AIDS could be traced to polio virus vaccines that were administered in the Belgian Congo between 1957 and 1960. The explanations behind this assertion were as follows: (1) All virus vaccines are made in cells; (2) the polio virus vaccine was grown in monkey kidney cells; (3) monkey kidney cells used at that time contained a virus (simian immunodeficiency virus, or SIV) similar to the virus that causes AIDS (human immunodeficiency virus, or HIV); and (4) people were inadvertently inoculated with SIV, which then mutated to HIV and caused the AIDS epidemic.

This reasoning is confounded by several false assumptions. First, although monkeys can be infected by SIV, a disease similar to HIV, SIV is not found in kidney cells. Second, SIV and HIV, although their spelling is very similar, are not genetically very close; mutation to one from the other would require centuries, not years. Third, SIV and HIV, although deadly viruses, are fairly fragile. Both of these viruses, if given by mouth (in a manner similar to the oral polio vaccine), would be rapidly destroyed by the enzymes and acids in the mouth and stomach. Last, original lots of the polio vaccine were recently tested for the presence of HIV using very sensitive tests that were not available in the late 1950s. These tests, called polymerase chain reaction, or PCR, are used today to diagnose HIV infection in children, adolescents, and adults. No HIV was present in any of those lots.

CONCERN: The polio virus vaccine is contaminated with a virus that causes cancer.

It is true that early lots of the polio vaccine used in the late 1950s and early 1960s were contaminated with a monkey virus called simian virus 40 or SV40. Recently, investigators found evidence for the presence of SV40 virus in a type of cancer called lymphoma. However, several facts should be noted. First, SV40 was present in cancers of people who either had or had not received the polio vaccine that was contaminated with SV40. Second, SV40 has not been present in any vaccine since the early 1960s. Third, people with lymphoma who were born after SV40 was no longer a contaminant of the polio vaccine were found to have evidence for SV40 in their cancerous cells. Taken together, these findings suggest that SV40 may be associated with some cancers, but that the virus is transmitted to people by a mechanism other than vaccines.

CONCERN: Vaccines may contain the agent that causes "mad-cow" disease.

On February 8, 2001, the *New York Times* published an article entitled "Five Drug Makers Use Material with Possible Mad-Cow Link." This article followed a Public Health Service statement on December 22,

2000, in *Morbidity and Mortality Weekly Report* (MMWR). MMWR is written by the CDC. The *New York Times* article and CDC report were prompted by the confluence of several events. First, as of July 2000, about 175,000 cows in the United Kingdom developed a disease called "mad-cow" disease—a progressive disease of the nervous system of cattle. Second, at least seventy-three people in the United Kingdom developed a progressive neurological disease called variant Creutzfeld-Jakob disease (vCJD) that may have resulted from eating meat prepared from cows with "mad-cow" disease. Third, some vaccines are made with serum or gelatin obtained from cows in England or from countries at risk for "mad-cow" disease.

What causes progressive neurological diseases such as "mad-cow" disease or vCJD?
vCJD is caused by an unusual protein called a prion (proteinaceous infectious particle). Prions are found in the brains of cows with "mad-cow" disease and in the brains of humans with vCJD. Prions can also be found in the spinal cord and in the back of the eye (retina).

However, blood from infected animals or blood from infected people has never been shown to be a source of infection to humans.

If prions are found only in the brain and spinal cord, why did people in England get vCJD after eating meat from cows?
The likely source of prions for people in England was hamburger, not steak, prepared from cows. Hamburger may be prepared in a manner that includes the spinal cord. Steak, on the other hand, represents only the muscles of cows and, therefore, does not contain prions.

Why do vaccines contain materials derived from cows?
Viral vaccines are weakened forms of natural viruses. Some viral vaccines are made by "growing" viruses in specialized cells in the laboratory. Many growth factors are needed for cells to grow. An excellent source of these growth factors is serum obtained from the fetuses of cows (known as fetal bovine serum). Fetal bovine serum is a naturally filtered source of growth factors. The natural filter is the bovine placenta. Whereas the human placenta contains one and a half layers that separate the mother's blood from fetal blood, the bovine

placenta contains six layers. Many proteins are excluded from the bovine fetal circulation by these six layers (for example, bovine fetal blood contains 1/500 of the antibodies found in bovine maternal blood).

Another product from animals (cows or pigs) that may be used in vaccines is gelatin. Gelatin is a protein formed by boiling skin or connective tissue (for example, hooves). Gelatin is used to stabilize vaccines so that they remain effective after manufacture.

Do vaccines that have been exposed to bovine materials during manufacture pose a risk for transmission of vCJD?
To answer this question, let's go through each step of the manufacturing process.

- Cows with "mad-cow" disease have prions in their brain, spinal cord, and retina. However, prions are not detected in their blood, skin, or connective tissue.

- Fetal bovine serum is used in the manufacture of vaccines. Fetal bovine serum is obtained from fetal blood, and blood is not a source of infection with prions. In addition, although cows "share" their blood with their unborn calves, the bovine placenta is a natural filter. Maternal-fetal transmission of prions has *never* been documented in animals.

- Fetal bovine serum is highly diluted and eventually removed from cells during the growth of vaccine viruses.

- Prions are propagated in mammalian brains and *not* in cell culture used to make vaccines. Therefore, prions are unlikely to be propagated in the cells used to grow vaccine viruses.

- Gelatin is also used in the manufacture of vaccines. Gelatin is added to vaccines at the end of the manufacturing process. However, gelatin is made from materials (skin and connective tissue) that do not contain prions. In addition, the preparation of gelatin often includes heat sterilization or treatment with organic solvents. It is likely that these treatments would inactivate prions.

- Transmission of prions occurs from either eating brains from infected animals or, in experimental studies, from directly inoculating preparations of brains from infected animals into the brains of experimental animals. Transmission of prions has *not* been documented after inoculation into the muscles or under the skin (routes used to vaccinate).

When you put all these factors together, the chance that currently licensed vaccines contain prions is essentially zero.

If vaccines pose no risk for progressive neurological diseases, why is the Public Health Service choosing to eventually eliminate bovine-derived materials obtained from countries at risk for "mad-cow" disease?
The Public Health Service is interested in maintaining the public's trust in immunizations. They are concerned that the public may fear that vaccines containing bovine material from countries at risk for "mad-cow" disease could potentially transmit this disease to children. So they have taken the precautionary steps of eventually eliminating the use of these materials in the production of vaccines. However, the facts about prion transmission should reassure us that it is essentially impossible for currently licensed vaccines to contain prions.

PART THREE

VACCINES FOR SOME CHILDREN AND ADULTS

CHAPTER 16

RABIES VACCINE

Will is seventeen years old. While in the backyard of a friend's house he is bitten on the hand by a cat. None of his friends ever saw the cat before, and it has not been seen since.

Should Will get the rabies vaccine?

Rabies is a uniformly fatal infection that is transmitted to people by the bite of a rabies-infected (or rabid) animal. Because people are occasionally bitten or scratched by animals, physicians and patients are commonly forced to decide about beginning a series of rabies shots.

The decision of whether to start this series of shots is a difficult one. Fortunately, however, it's not as hard as it used to be. Before 1980, rabies immunization meant a series of up to thirty shots given in the skin over the abdomen. This was often a painful and frightening experience for children and parents. Also, the vaccine didn't always work. About 20 percent of those immunized were not protected against rabies.

Today rabies immunization consists of a series of five shots given in the shoulder muscle, and the vaccine is completely protective and very safe. In this chapter we talk about who should get the rabies vaccine and why.

**Recommendation by the American
Academy of Pediatrics**

Treatment of children bitten by an animal likely to transmit rabies consists of the following three things:
1. Washing the wound carefully with soap and water.
2. Administering a shot of rabies immune globulin.
3. Giving a rabies vaccine at the time of exposure and then three, seven, fourteen, and twenty-eight days after exposure (a total of five shots). Shots are given in the shoulder muscle.

WHAT IS RABIES?

Rabies is a virus that infects the brain and nervous system and, because virtually no one survives infection, is one of the most feared diseases. It is transmitted to humans from the bite of an infected animal.

The disease usually begins with indistinct symptoms such as fatigue, sore throat, chills, vomiting, and headache. After about one week, symptoms include hallucinations, bizarre behavior, disorientation, hyperactivity, and the inability to swallow. Progression to paralysis, coma, and death is inevitable.

Although cases of rabies in developed countries have received intensive medical support, only three people are known to have ever survived.

**Rabies Vaccine Works Even
after Exposure to Rabies**

The rabies vaccine is unusual in that it works even after someone is infected with the virus. Rabies has a long incubation period (the time from exposure to development of symptoms). Whereas diseases such as influenza have incubation periods as short as one or two days, the average incubation period for rabies is about two months. This means that after a bite from an infected animal there is still plenty of time (before symptoms appear) to develop protective immunity from the vaccine.

WHAT IS THE RABIES VACCINE?

The rabies virus normally grows in cells of the human nervous system. The rabies vaccine was made by taking rabies virus from the nervous system of an infected person and adapting it to growth in specialized cells grown in the laboratory. The cells in which rabies virus was grown were human lung cells (the vaccine is also called the human diploid cell vaccine, or HDCV). The rabies vaccine is also grown in chick embryo cells. To make a vaccine, rabies virus was grown in these cells, purified, and inactivated with a chemical (β-propiolactone). Because the rabies virus can't replicate, it is called a killed, or inactivated, vaccine.

More than 500 people bitten by animals proven to be infected with rabies have received rabies vaccine. None of these people got rabies. Therefore, the vaccine, if used correctly, appears to be 100 percent effective.

The First Rabies Vaccine

The rabies vaccine was developed by Louis Pasteur in the late nineteenth century. An account of the first child to receive the vaccine follows:

"Mrs. Meister from Meissnegott in Alsace . . . came crying into the laboratory, leading her 9-year-old boy, Joseph, gashed in fourteen places two days before by a mad dog. He was a pitifully whimpering, scared boy—hardly able to walk.

" 'Save my little boy—Mr. Pasteur,' this woman begged him. . . .

"And that night of July 6, 1885, they made the first injection of the weakened microbes of hydrophobia [rabies] into a human being. Then, day after day, the boy Meister went without a hitch through his fourteen injections—which were only slight pricks of the hypodermic needle into his skin.

"And the boy went home to Alsace and had never a sign of that dreadful disease."

Paul de Kruif, *Microbe Hunters*, 1926

Doesn't the rabies vaccine mean getting many painful shots?

The rabies vaccine used in this country until 1980 had some problems. The virus was grown in cells from duck eggs (called duck embryo vaccine, or DEV) and had a fairly high rate of side effects.

The DEV was given as a series of twenty-three to thirty shots in the skin over the abdomen. Even after this torturous experience, up to 20 percent of children were not protected against rabies. The DEV is no longer available in the United States and has been replaced by safer vaccines.

Who should get the rabies vaccine?

The rabies vaccine should be given to anyone who is exposed to an animal likely to have rabies.

What counts as an exposure?

Rabies can be transmitted by a bite or a nonbite exposure from a rabid animal. A bite means that the animal's teeth have penetrated the child's skin. A nonbite means that a rabid animal has licked an open wound, a scratch, a cut, or a mucous membrane (such as the mouth, nose, or eyes). Therefore, petting a rabid animal would not be considered an exposure.

What animals are likely to have rabies?

The animals likely to have rabies are determined by the area in which you live. Therefore, the smartest thing a person can do after an animal bite is to call the local health department and find out whether a particular species of animal in that area is likely to be rabid. A few general rules can be reassuring in the meantime:

1. Because most dogs and cats in the United States get a rabies vaccine, it is uncommon for them to catch or transmit rabies. If a person is bitten by a dog or cat, the animal should be observed for ten days. If the animal acts normally (doesn't show signs of rabies), there is no need for the vaccine. If the animal cannot be observed, then the vaccine should begin as outlined above.

2. Animals such as mice, rats, squirrels, rabbits, birds, chipmunks, or reptiles rarely, if ever, transmit rabies.

3. The animals most likely to transmit rabies in the United States are raccoons, skunks, foxes, and bats. Treatment should usually be given after bites from any of these animals.

Is the rabies vaccine safe?

More than 1 million doses of the rabies vaccine have been given, and the vaccine is safe. Even infants may receive it, if necessary.

However, the vaccine does have a fairly high rate of *mild* side effects. Some people who receive the rabies vaccine develop a sore arm (15 to 25 percent), headache (5 to 8 percent), or nausea (2 to 5 percent).

The rabies vaccine is also associated with allergic reactions. After the first dose, several cases of anaphylaxis characterized by swelling of the mouth or throat, low blood pressure, or hives (0.1 percent) have been reported. In addition, the incidence of anaphylaxis from subsequent, or booster, doses of the rabies vaccine can be as high as 6 percent. There has not been a fatality caused by modern rabies vaccines.

Can you get rabies from the rabies vaccine?

Because the rabies virus in the vaccine is inactivated, it is not possible to get rabies from the vaccine.

RABIES VACCINE: SUMMARY AND CONCLUSIONS

Rabies is caused by a virus transmitted by the bite of a rabid animal. Because people are occasionally bitten or scratched by animals potentially infected with rabies, a decision must be made as to whether to begin the series of rabies shots. Before 1980, the decision of whether to begin a series of rabies shots was hard; the "old" vaccine involved a series of twenty-three to thirty shots, didn't always work, and had a fairly high rate of side effects. These days the decision is easier; the current rabies vaccine is safer, is virtually 100 percent effective, and involves a series of only five shots.

INFLUENZA VACCINE ("THE FLU SHOT")

Sarah is three years old. It seems that every time she gets a cold she wheezes. About six months ago, Sarah had an episode in which the wheezing was so bad that she had to see the doctor in the emergency room. The doctor says that Sarah has asthma and that she will probably grow out of it.

Sarah's mother has heard that children who have asthma may benefit from getting the influenza vaccine. Is this true?

Influenza, or flu, is a highly contagious viral illness that causes high fever, muscle aches, and coughing. Some children and adults are at risk of getting severe or fatal pneumonia from influenza.

Children at risk of contracting severe influenza disease should get the influenza vaccine. For example, the vaccine is recommended for use in all children with asthma. Further, the influenza vaccine should be given to any person living in the home of someone with asthma.

Unfortunately, the vaccine is not often given to those who really need it, and it is probably the most underused vaccine in pediatrics.

Recently, the Centers for Disease Control and Prevention (CDC) stated that *all* infants and young children six to twenty-three months of age should be "encouraged" to receive the influenza vaccine.

The influenza vaccine is unusual in that it is given every year. This is because the influenza viruses that cause disease one year are often different from those that cause it the following year.

In this chapter we discuss who should get the influenza vaccine and why.

Recommendation by the American Academy of Pediatrics

Children older than six months of age who are at risk for severe influenza infection (see the list below) should receive the influenza vaccine *every fall*. If the child is receiving influenza vaccine for the first time and is between six months and eight years of age, the vaccine is given as two shots one month apart. If the child is nine years old or older, the first dose of the vaccine is given as a single shot.

In addition, both the AAP and the CDC recently recommended that *all* infants and young children six to twenty-three months of age be "encouraged" to receive the influenza vaccine.

All subsequent, yearly doses of vaccine are given as a single shot.

WHAT IS INFLUENZA?

Influenza, or flu, is a virus that infects the windpipe (trachea) and breathing tubes (bronchi). The illness usually begins with high fever, chills, severe muscle aches, and headache. These symptoms are so severe that patients usually remember the exact hour when the illness began.

As the fever and muscle aches subside, the patient develops a runny nose, cough, and sometimes a feeling of burning in the chest. These symptoms are caused by the destruction of the lining of the trachea and bronchi. The cough can last as long as one to two weeks.

Up to 25 percent of people develop complications from influenza. These complications include severe pneumonia or worsening of asthma.

Influenza Causes Epidemics and Pandemics

Epidemics are outbreaks of an infection confined to a specific location (such as a town, city, or country). Influenza epidemics occur every one to three years in the United States and kill about 20,000 people yearly.

Each century, influenza causes about eight pandemics (outbreaks of disease that occur worldwide). The worst pandemic in recent history occurred between 1918 and 1919, when 550,000 people were killed in the United States and 21 million people were killed throughout the world by influenza.

WHAT IS THE INFLUENZA VACCINE?

The influenza virus normally grows in cells that line the windpipe (trachea) and breathing tubes (bronchi). The influenza vaccine is made by taking influenza viruses from the throats of infected children and adapting them to grow in chicken embryos (eggs). The virus is then harvested from the eggs, purified, and inactivated with formaldehyde. The vaccine contains the three strains of influenza that are likely to cause infection that year.

Because the influenza virus in the vaccine cannot replicate, it is called a killed, or inactivated, vaccine.

Is the influenza vaccine safe?

Fever, muscle aches, and malaise occur in less than 1 percent of those who receive the influenza vaccine. These side effects usually begin six to twelve hours after vaccination and can persist for one to two days. Side effects are most likely to occur in those who were never before infected with influenza virus or never immunized with influenza vaccine (usually younger children).

The Great Epidemic

"By December of that year of mingled victory and catastrophe, 1918, five hundred thousand Americans had perished in a great plague, and nearly 20 million had sickened. The world had never in history been ravaged by a killer that slew so many human beings so quickly, during a few weeks in autumn.

"This microscopic marauder that could not be seen, heard, or even sensed, and was infinitely more deadly than any weapon from the crucible of the World War, was labeled, almost beguilingly, 'Spanish influenza.'"

A. A. Hoehling, *The Great Epidemic,* 1961

Sometimes people who have symptoms of fever, muscle aches, and malaise claim that they "got the flu" from the influenza vaccine. However, because the influenza virus in the vaccine is inactivated, it cannot cause the respiratory symptoms or pneumonia commonly seen in influenza infections.

In rare instances, immediate allergic reactions (hives, swelling of the throat, low blood pressure, or shock) occur after getting the influenza vaccine. These reactions are probably caused by allergies to the residual egg proteins in the vaccine. For this reason, *people with severe allergy to eggs generally are advised not to receive the influenza vaccine.* However, for those people who are at great risk for severe influenza disease (such as those with asthma), there are methods to desensitize the person to the vaccine prior to administration.

Who should get the influenza vaccine?

The influenza vaccine should be given to all children and adults at high risk of getting severe pneumonia from influenza infection. *In addition, the influenza vaccine should be given to anyone living in the home of someone at high risk.* Several diseases, listed on the next page, are considered to put people at high risk of severe pneumonia.

1. Asthma

2. Diabetes

3. Heart disease

4. Kidney disease

5. Sickle cell disease

6. Cystic fibrosis

7. Lung disease of prematurity (called bronchopulmonary dysplasia, or BPD)

8. AIDS or HIV infection

9. Cancer, lymphoma, or leukemia

10. Long-term aspirin therapy

Recently, the CDC and AAP changed their policies to recommend that *all* children six to twenty-three months of age be "encouraged" to use the influenza vaccine, rather than only those children at high-risk of complications from influenza.

Why did the CDC and AAP change their policies? While every year about 20,000 people in the United States die from pneumonia caused by influenza virus (most of these deaths occur in people over fifty years of age), the group *most* likely to be hospitalized by influenza infections are children less than one year of age! Infants hospitalized with influenza usually have pneumonia, fever, wheezing, or cough. Most of these hospitalized infants were previously healthy and were not in the high-risk groups listed above.

Because the influenza vaccine is given seasonally (in the late fall and early winter), and because two additional shots will be added to an already-crowded immunization schedule, it may be difficult for doctors to give the influenza vaccine to all young children. However, its benefits are clear. Recent studies that immunization of previously healthy infants and young children with influenza vaccine not only decreased the incidence of influenza hospitalization in those children, but also decreased hospitalizations of adults who were in contact with those children.

Influenza Is Very Contagious

Up to 40 percent of people exposed to influenza will get sick.

Isn't there a new influenza vaccine given to children as nose drops?

An influenza vaccine that is given as a nasal spray is currently being developed. This vaccine is not yet licensed in the United States but has been tested in infants, children, and adults with very promising results. The vaccine should be licensed soon. Because the vaccine is effective and easy to administer, it is likely that it would be recommended for *all* infants and young children, not just those at high risk of severe disease.

The "nasal-spray" influenza vaccine will be enormously useful. Because the vaccine is not given as a series of shots, it can be administered to all young infants without burdening an already crowded immunization schedule.

The Swine Flu

In 1976, public health officials discovered something alarming. In Fort Dix, New Jersey, an outbreak of influenza virus infection in military recruits was caused by a strain (called "swine flu") very different from other circulating strains.

These strains often herald the beginning of influenza pandemics. Public health officials decided to immunize everyone in the country to prevent a nationwide outbreak.

Didn't the "swine flu" vaccine cause paralysis in some people?

The "swine flu" vaccine was administered in the United States in a mass immunization program in 1976 and was associated with a disease called Guillain-Barré syndrome in about one in 200,000 vaccine recipients. People with Guillain-Barré syndrome developed paralysis that began in the legs and spread to the arms and breathing muscles. Most people recovered without permanent damage.

Since 1976, millions of adults and children have been immunized with the influenza vaccine. If the current influenza vaccine is a cause of Guillain-Barré syndrome (an association that is unproven), it does so at a rate of fewer than one case per 1,000,000 doses. The reasons for the association between "swine flu" vaccine and Guillain-Barré syndrome remain unclear.

INFLUENZA VACCINE: SUMMARY AND CONCLUSIONS

Influenza virus is an unusual cause of death in otherwise healthy young children. However, healthy children are commonly hospitalized when the influenza virus causes fever, croup, bronchitis, or pneumonia. Because the vaccine does not cause serious reactions, the benefits of the vaccine clearly outweigh its risks in *all* young children.

CHAPTER 18

MENINGOCOCCAL VACCINE ("THE SEPSIS/MENINGITIS VACCINE")

Amy is fourteen years old. One day after school, she tells her mother that one of her classmates was in the hospital with meningitis. Two days later, Amy's mother discovers that the classmate has died of the disease.

Is there a chance that Amy caught meningitis from her classmate?

Are vaccines available that could prevent Amy from getting meningitis?

No infectious disease is more terrifying to parents than that caused by meningococcus.

A healthy child can progress from a mild rash and fever to shock, coma, and death within twelve hours. When meningococcus enters a child-care center or school, the panic that spreads through a community is unlike that caused by any other illness.

Like pneumococcus and Hib, meningococcus usually infects children under four years of age. The next groups most likely to get the disease are older adolescents and college freshmen. Unfortunately, an effective vaccine for meningococcus has been difficult to develop for young children. Therefore, the meningococcal vaccine is used primarily for children older than two years of age at particularly high risk of infection.

In this chapter we discuss who should get the meningococcal vaccine, whether the vaccine should be used during community outbreaks of infection or on college campuses, and the prospects for a better vaccine.

Recommendation by the American Academy of Pediatrics

The meningococcal vaccine is recommended for children older than two years of age at high risk for getting severe meningococcal disease (see below). The vaccine is also recommended to be considered for all incoming college freshmen.

The vaccine is given as a single shot.

WHAT IS MENINGOCOCCUS?

Meningococcus is a bacterium (*Neisseria meningitidis*) that is a common cause of sepsis (a bloodstream infection) and meningitis (infection of the lining of the brain) in children under four years of age. Every year in the United States, meningococcus causes about 3,000 cases of sepsis and meningitis.

The sepsis caused by meningococcus is often rapid and overwhelming. Healthy children can progress from a mild rash and fever to shock, coma, and death within twelve hours. Despite a quick medical response and appropriate therapy, as many as 30 percent of children with sepsis will die from the infection.

Children with meningitis caused by meningococcus often have symptoms similar to those with Hib: high fever, headache, drowsiness, and a stiff neck. About one in twenty children with meningococcal meningitis will die, and many of those who survive will be left with brain damage.

Epidemics of Meningococcus Happen Every Year

Every year in the United States, epidemics of sepsis and meningitis caused by meningococcus occur in child-care centers and schools.

WHAT IS THE MENINGOCOCCAL VACCINE?

Meningococcus is similar to both pneumococcus and Hib. All three bacteria are coated with polysaccharide (a sugar). Protection against disease is caused by antibodies directed against this sugar. Unfortunately, infants and children under two years of age can't develop immunity to this sugar.

Researchers found that if sugars are joined to harmless proteins, producing conjugate vaccines, younger children could make antibodies to the sugars. Unfortunately, the current meningococcal vaccine is unconjugated and consists only of the sugar.

There are at least five different types of meningococcus (types A, B, C, Y, and W-135). It is very difficult to make a vaccine against one meningococcal type—type B—which causes about half of the meningococcus outbreaks. Therefore, the current meningococcal vaccine contains only types A, C, Y, and W-135.

Is the meningococcal vaccine safe?

Yes. There are no serious side effects from the vaccine. However, the meningococcal vaccine does cause pain or soreness where the shot is given in about 4 percent of children.

Who should get the meningococcal vaccine?

The meningococcal vaccine should be given to children over two years of age who are at high risk of getting meningococcal infection. This includes children with the following very unusual problems or situations:

1. Absence of a spleen, as with children who have had their spleens removed following trauma.

2. Lack of a specific group of serum proteins (called complement proteins) that help the body fight infection.

3. Travel to sub-Saharan Africa during the dry season (December through June).

In addition, the vaccine should be given to all incoming college freshmen.

If the diseases caused by meningococcus are so bad, why not give the vaccine to all children?

The meningococcal vaccine has been hard to develop. To make a successful vaccine, researchers have tried to overcome two obstacles. First, they have tried to devise a way to link all five types of meningococcus to proteins and put them in a single conjugate vaccine. Although it is likely that this can be achieved for four of the five types of meningococcus, it is not likely that this will be achieved for meningococcus type B.

The second and more difficult task is to find a way to get both children and adults to successfully respond to type B, the type that causes about half of all meningococcal disease. Meningococcus type B shares a substance called neuraminic acid that is identical to one on the surface of some fetal nervous system cells. Therefore, girls or women vaccinated against meningococcus type B (a type *not* included in the current vaccine) may inadvertently make antibodies directed against their future unborn child. This could have disastrous effects and may forever preclude the development of a vaccine that uses the sugar of meningococcus type B. However, researchers have now identified a protein of type B meningococcus that might serve as an effective vaccine.

Until these significant problems in vaccine development are solved, younger children will continue to die from sepsis and meningitis caused by this bacterium.

Recently two children in my son's school had meningitis. The public health officer said that these children were infected with meningococcus. What should I do?

If your child is exposed to a child in school who has meningitis caused by meningococcus, two things should be done.

First, an antibiotic (rifampin or ciprofloxacin) is recommended for those children who either live in the home of an infected person or attend the same child-care center or nursery school. *In elementary school or high school, one is considered to be exposed if the contact is intimate (meaning kissing or sharing food or beverages). Otherwise, children in school, church, or community center settings do not need antibiotics.*

Second, if an outbreak of meningitis in a school is caused by a type of meningococcus that is contained in the vaccine (type A, C, Y, or W-135), the vaccine might help protect children from getting infected. Parents should try to find out what type of bacteria is causing the outbreak of sepsis or meningitis in the child's school or day-care center and follow the recommendations of local public health authorities.

If a child in school has meningitis caused by pneumococcus, neither antibiotics nor vaccines are recommended, because the risk of a spread to other children is so low.

Does the meningococcus vaccine protect against meningitis?

No. The meningococcus vaccine protects against one type of bacterial meningitis. Two other bacteria cause bacterial meningitis. One, Hib, is now successfully controlled by a vaccine first available in 1990. The other, pneumonococcus, will probably be controlled by a vaccine first available in 2000. So, the meningococcus vaccine protects against one important type of bacterial meningitis, but not all bacterial meningitis.

My daughter is a freshman in college. She was recently told that she should consider getting the meningococcal vaccine. Is this really necessary?

Between 1980 and 1993, one outbreak of meningitis caused by meningococcus occurred on a college campus. An outbreak was defined as more than five cases caused by the same strain of meningococcus within a three-month period. Recently, however, those statistics have changed dramatically. Over the past ten years, at least six outbreaks have occurred on college campuses. Although meningococcus remains a problem primarily of young children, it seems that young adults living on campus may be at greater risk now than they were before. For this reason, the meningococcal vaccine should be given to all incoming college freshmen living on campus.

MENINGOCOCCAL VACCINE: SUMMARY AND CONCLUSIONS

Every year in the United States, meningococcus causes thousands of cases of sepsis and meningitis in children under four years of age. Many of these children die or are left permanently disabled by these infections. Unfortunately, the current meningococcal vaccine is not very effective in preventing disease in younger children. Therefore, the vaccine is recommended only for those at particularly high risk of disease. The meningococcal vaccine is likely to be of value in community outbreaks of infection and for all young adults living on college campuses.

CHAPTER 19

TUBERCULOSIS VACCINE

Christopher is six years old. Christopher's mother learns that a seventy-two-year-old uncle, who had seen Christopher at a party three weeks ago, has tuberculosis.

What should Christopher's mother do? Is there a vaccine to prevent tuberculosis?

Tuberculosis has had a recent resurgence in this country. Although the incidence of the disease steadily declined between 1950 and 1984, the incidence has steadily risen between 1985 and 1991. During that period, there were about 40,000 more cases than would have been predicted. The single most important reason for the increase in tuberculosis is the introduction of the AIDS virus into the United States. People with AIDS are at high risk of developing tuberculosis and spreading it to others.

Because the number of people with tuberculosis is increasing, and because children are now at increased risk of catching the disease, the Centers for Disease Control and Prevention recently reconsidered its policy on the tuberculosis vaccine. The results of that decision are described below.

Recommendation by the Centers for Disease Control and Prevention

The tuberculosis vaccine is recommended only for children who live in very unusual situations. Children are recommended to receive the vaccine if they are in the same household as someone actively infected with tuberculosis who either (1) cannot take the antibiotics that treat tuberculosis or (2) is infected with a strain of the tuberculosis bacteria that is highly resistant to antibiotics. This situation applies only to a very small number of children in this country.

WHAT IS TUBERCULOSIS?

Tuberculosis is a disease caused by a bacterium called *Mycobacterium tuberculosis*. This bacterium can infect every organ of the body, but most prominently infects the lungs.

People with tuberculosis infection of the lungs usually have a persistent, unrelenting cough. Occasionally the sputum brought up by the cough is streaked with blood. The patient also can develop sweating at night, loss of weight, and a progressive decrease in physical activity. If left untreated, the disease is often fatal (in the old days tuberculosis was called "consumption").

Children under five years of age will occasionally get a very severe form of tuberculosis associated with meningitis or a rapid, overwhelming, often fatal form of infection called "miliary" tuberculosis.

Many people become infected with tuberculosis without knowing it. They don't develop any symptoms of tuberculosis when they are first infected. However, as they get older, the bacteria can reawaken, or reactivate, and cause severe lung disease. The way to tell whether someone is infected is to do a skin test called PPD. Children living in or around an area where tuberculosis is present are usually tested two or three times by five years of age to see whether they have been exposed to tuberculosis.

> ## The Impact of Tuberculosis
>
> Tuberculosis kills more people in the world than any other infection. It currently infects 1.7 billion people worldwide, about one-third of the world's population.

WHAT IS THE TUBERCULOSIS VACCINE?

Many parents are surprised to hear that there is a tuberculosis vaccine.

The tuberculosis vaccine is called BCG, which stands for Bacillus of Calmette and Guérin. It has been given to billions of people. Since the 1960s, the only countries that have *not* routinely used the BCG vaccine are the United States and the Netherlands.

The BCG vaccine is made from a bacterium (called *Mycobacterium bovis*) that was originally isolated from cows by two French scientists, Calmette and Guérin, in 1908. The researchers reasoned that the cow tuberculosis bacterium was similar enough to the human tuberculosis bacterium that immunization with one would protect against disease caused by the other. They weakened this bovine tuberculosis strain by continually growing it in a nutrient broth for a period of thirteen years.

In 1921, the vaccine was first used in humans. For the most part, the vaccine is not effective in preventing adolescents and adults from getting the lung disease caused by tuberculosis. However, it is effective about 80 percent of the time in preventing young children from getting the severe form of tuberculosis (meaning tuberculous meningitis or rapid, overwhelming tuberculosis infection).

Is the tuberculosis vaccine safe?

The tuberculosis vaccine is safe. About three out of every 10,000 children less than one year of age will develop a painful swelling of the glands under the arm that was injected with the vaccine. This swelling can last as long as three months.

How do you catch tuberculosis?

Tuberculosis can be very contagious. The disease is spread by tiny droplets produced by coughing, sneezing, or even talking. Up to 3,000 infectious droplets can be produced after one cough, one sneeze, or talking for about five minutes.

Two outbreaks of tuberculosis in closed environments show just how contagious the disease can be. One person on the submarine *Byrd* infected 45 percent of the entire crew. An elderly man in a nursing home infected about 80 percent of the residents living in the same wing.

Who should get the tuberculosis vaccine?

The United States is trying to stop the spread of tuberculosis by treating with antibiotics those people who have disease of the lungs or who are silently infected with the bacteria. The hope is that vigorous identification of these infections and treatment with appropriate antibiotics will prevent the spread of tuberculosis. Because the vaccine is not effective in preventing infections in the lungs of adolescents and adults, BCG vaccine is not routinely used in the United States.

The vaccine is recommended only for children living in very unusual situations. Children are recommended to receive the vaccine if they are in the same household as someone who is actively infected with tuberculosis and either (1) cannot take the antibiotics that treat tuberculosis or (2) is infected with a strain of bacteria that is very resistant to antibiotics. This situation currently applies to only a very small number of children in this country.

What are we doing about tuberculosis in this country?

The United States uses two approaches to eliminate tuberculosis.

First, it seeks to eliminate the possibilities for spreading the disease by identifying people who are actively infected with tuberculosis and treating them with appropriate antibiotics. Although people who have severe tuberculosis infection of the lungs are very contagious, treatment with antibiotics (such as isoniazid [INH], rifampin, ethambutal, or pyrazinamide) stops the shedding of bacteria within two weeks.

Second, the United States tries to identify people who are silently infected with the tuberculosis bacterium and treat them with antibiotics. People who are silently infected have a positive skin test (PPD) but no symptoms. Treating them with antibiotics such as INH makes it much less likely that the bacteria will reactivate and later cause disease of the lungs or other organs.

TUBERCULOSIS VACCINE: SUMMARY AND CONCLUSIONS

The tuberculosis vaccine is not very good at preventing infection of the lungs in teenagers and adults. Therefore, it is not routinely used in this country. However, because of the resurgence of tuberculosis in the United States, the vaccine is now recommended in certain unusual situations. The tuberculosis vaccine is recommended for children who live in the same household as someone who has tuberculosis infection of the lungs if the infected person either can't take antibiotics or is infected with a strain of tuberculosis that is highly resistant to antibiotics.

PART FOUR

VACCINES FOR TRAVELERS

CHAPTER 20

SOURCES OF INFORMATION ABOUT VACCINES FOR TRAVELERS

In August of 1996, a Tennessee man came back from a fishing trip in South America and died of yellow fever. He was the first person to die of this disease in the United States in over seventy years. Although he knew that the yellow fever vaccine was recommended for travel to the Amazon Basin, he had chosen not to get it.

Traveling to other countries occasionally exposes one to microorganisms that are rarely, if ever, encountered in the United States. Many of these microorganisms are potentially deadly. Unfortunately, many travelers don't know how to find out about the diseases that are prevalent in different countries or about the vaccines available to prevent them. It is especially difficult to determine which vaccines can be taken safely by young children. Although travel agents and airlines are willing to inform traveler's about vaccines *required* for travel, rarely do they inform travelers about vaccines that are *recommended* for travel.

So how can you get this information?

First, there are many travel clinics in this country that provide information about infectious diseases in different parts of the world and the vaccines that prevent them. One can usually find out about the availability of these clinics from travel agents, doctors, or medical centers.

Second, a book published by the Centers for Disease Control and Prevention (CDC) called *Health Information for International Travel* is available for sale from the Superintendent of Documents, Government Printing Office, Washington, DC 20402; (202) 512-1800. Unfortunately, patterns of diseases, especially in developing countries, can change fairly rapidly, and information in books can lose relevance.

Third, the CDC maintains a web site that constantly updates information on vaccines both recommended and required for travel (http://www.cdc.gov).

Finally, the CDC has an updated voice information service at 1-877-394-8747.

Many people who travel don't understand the difference between vaccines that are "required" and those that are "recommended." Most people believe that a vaccine is required to prevent disease from a likely exposure, and that a vaccine is recommended to prevent disease from an unlikely exposure. This interpretation is almost the exact opposite of the truth.

Vaccines are required because a country does not want its own citizens exposed to a particular disease. The requirement is an attempt to limit the importation of that disease into the country. In contrast, vaccines are recommended when a disease is prevalent in a country and the *visitors'* risk of exposure is high. To put it another way, required vaccines protect the people in the country you are visiting and recommended vaccines protect you, the visitor.

The chapters that follow contain detailed descriptions of five vaccines used to prevent some of the diseases highly prevalent abroad: hepatitis A virus, cholera, typhoid, yellow fever, and Japanese encephalitis virus. It should also be noted that children *and* adults should be up to date on the eleven vaccines that are universally recommended (measles, mumps, rubella, polio, diphtheria, pertussis, tetanus, hepatitis B, Hib, pneumococcus, and varicella).

CHAPTER 21

HEPATITIS A VACCINE

Karen and Andrew are traveling to Jamaica and want to take three-year-old Fred with them. They will be going to places in Jamaica with standard tourist accommodations and food.

Are there any vaccines that Fred should get before he leaves?

Hepatitis A virus is a common cause of hepatitis (inflammation of the liver). In the United States about 100,000 cases of hepatitis A occur every year. In developing countries in Asia, Africa, South America, Central America, the Caribbean, southern Europe, the Middle East (including Israel), the Mediterranean Basin, and Mexico the disease is common. Almost *all* adults living in developing countries have been infected at some time in their lives with hepatitis A virus.

A vaccine to prevent hepatitis A virus was licensed by the Food and Drug Administration in February of 1995. Because the virus is so prevalent in many areas of the world, all travelers to developing countries (even those using standard tourist accommodations, itineraries, and food) should receive the hepatitis A vaccine. Hepatitis A virus infection is the most common vaccine-preventable disease in travelers.

Recommendation by the American Academy of Pediatrics and the CDC

The hepatitis A virus vaccine is recommended for travel to *all* countries *except* Australia, Canada, Japan, New Zealand, Scandinavia, and countries in western Europe. Travelers to all other countries (including Mexico and the Caribbean) should receive the vaccine.

The vaccine is given to children at least two years of age in the form of two shots. The second shot is given six to twelve months after the first.

WHAT IS HEPATITIS A?

Hepatitis A is a virus that causes hepatitis, or inflammation of the liver. Children and adults usually have fever, yellowing of the skin (jaundice), loss of appetite, nausea, and vomiting. Hepatitis A virus infections are much less severe than hepatitis B virus infections and are rarely a cause of death or permanent liver damage.

WHAT IS THE HEPATITIS A VACCINE?

The hepatitis A vaccine contains the whole virus that is killed by treatment with the chemical formaldehyde. Because the virus cannot replicate, it cannot cause hepatitis.

Is the hepatitis A vaccine safe?

Although it is relatively new, hundreds of thousands of people have been given the hepatitis A vaccine without any serious side effects. About 5 to 10 percent of vaccine recipients will have pain, warmth, or swelling where the shot was given and about 5 percent will have a headache.

In which countries can you catch hepatitis A?

Outbreaks of hepatitis A can occur in any country in the world. However, the disease is most prevalent in Asia, Africa, South America, Central

America, the Middle East, the Mediterranean Basin, southern Europe, the Caribbean, and Mexico.

How can I avoid catching hepatitis A virus?

In developing countries, hepatitis A virus is transmitted by contaminated food or water. Travelers can best avoid catching the virus by avoiding uncooked shellfish, uncooked or peeled fruits or vegetables, beverages with ice, or water of unknown purity.

Unfortunately, many persons catch hepatitis A virus while traveling to countries where the disease is prevalent despite standard tourist accommodations, itineraries, and foods. Therefore, the vaccine is recommended for *all* persons traveling to those countries.

Why Shellfish Contain Hepatitis A Virus

To obtain adequate quantities of food, shellfish (such as oysters, mussels, clams, crabs, and lobsters) filter hundreds of quarts of water every day. Hepatitis A virus (present in the water) is concentrated in the shellfish.

Is the hepatitis A virus vaccine required for international travel?

The hepatitis A virus vaccine is not required for international travel, but it is *recommended* for adults and *all* children over two years of age who are traveling to countries where the disease is highly prevalent.

I am going to Mexico with my five-year-old son, and we are leaving in one week. Do I have enough time to get my son vaccinated with the hepatitis A vaccine?

A period of at least four weeks is required for about 90 percent of children to become protected against disease after getting the vaccine. Therefore, parents should make every effort to give their children the vaccine at least four weeks before traveling. However, many children are probably protected against hepatitis A virus infection within two weeks of the first dose of vaccine. So it is still worth getting the hepatitis A vaccine even if you know you are traveling within two weeks.

To ensure protection against hepatitis A virus for children or adults whose travel is imminent (meaning within four weeks), it is also of value to inject immunoglobulin (antibodies directed against hepatitis A virus) at the same time that the vaccine is given. Unfortunately, the national supply of immunoglobulin is low. Because of this shortage, it is now more important than ever to get the hepatitis A vaccine well before departure.

For long-term protection against hepatitis A virus infection (at least ten years), two shots are required.

I am traveling to Nassau in the Bahamas with my daughter, who is only fifteen months old. Is she too young to get the hepatitis A vaccine?

The hepatitis A vaccine is not recommended for children under two years of age. Parents traveling to areas where hepatitis A virus is prevalent (including the Bahamas) should ask their doctor to give their child a single shot of immunoglobulin, antibodies directed against hepatitis A virus, prior to travel. The immunoglobulin will protect the child against infection with hepatitis A virus for up to three months.

Does hepatitis A virus cause disease in the United States?

Unfortunately, hepatitis A virus still infects tens of thousands of people every year in the United States. Many of these cases occur in children and about 100 people die from the disease. Some areas of the country are at particularly high risk. In these states the rate of infection is at least two times the national average. States with a relatively high rate of hepatitis A virus infections include Alaska, Arizona, California, Idaho, Nevada, New Mexico, Oklahoma, Oregon, South Dakota, Utah, and Washington. The Centers for Disease Control and Prevention (CDC) now recommends that all children living in states with a high risk of hepatitis A virus infection be vaccinated with hepatitis A vaccine. However, because hepatitis A virus infections occur to some extent throughout the United States, there probably will be a time when the hepatitis A vaccine is recommended routinely for all children in this country.

In addition to travelers, who else is at risk of catching hepatitis A virus?

Several different groups of people are at relatively high risk of catching hepatitis A virus infection. Groups include adults who work in day-care centers, injecting drug users, men who have sex with men, hemophilia patients, and people with long-term (chronic) liver disease. These groups should be vaccinated with the hepatitis A vaccine.

HEPATITIS A VACCINE: SUMMARY AND CONCLUSIONS

Hepatitis A virus is a common cause of hepatitis worldwide. Although the disease is rarely fatal, symptoms can be quite disabling.

Hepatitis A virus is so prevalent worldwide that it is easier to list countries where you don't need the vaccine than those where you do need it. Children over two years of age traveling to *all* countries *except* Australia, Canada, Japan, New Zealand, Scandinavia, and countries in western Europe should receive the vaccine.

In addition, all children living in states with a relatively high risk of hepatitis A virus infection should be vaccinated with the hepatitis A vaccine.

CHAPTER 22

CHOLERA VACCINE

Kurt and Adele are planning a trip to India. They have read in newspapers that there are outbreaks of cholera in India.

Is there a cholera vaccine? If so, should they get the vaccine?

Cholera is a cause of severe diarrhea and water loss, or dehydration, in India, Southeast Asia, Africa, the Middle East, southern Europe, the western Pacific Islands (Oceania), South America, and some parts of central Asia. Every year more than one million people are infected and about 100,000 die from cholera. Most of these cases occur in Asia and Africa.

Travelers using standard tourist accommodations to areas where cholera is prevalent are at virtually no risk of disease.

No country requires the cholera vaccine for entry.

Two cholera vaccines are made outside the United States: one in Sweden, the other in Switzerland. However, neither of these vaccines is recommended for travelers and both are unavailable in the United States.

Recommendation by the American Academy of Pediatrics and the CDC

The cholera vaccine is not required for entry into any country, nor is it recommended for those who stay in standard tourist accommodations in areas where the disease is prevalent. The cholera vaccine is not available in the United States.

WHAT IS CHOLERA?

Cholera is a bacterium (*Vibrio cholera*) that infects the intestines. Most people infected with cholera have no symptoms, but some (about 5 percent) have severe diarrhea. The diarrhea caused by cholera can be so severe that a person can go into shock within four hours of the beginning of illness.

A Death in Venice

"For several years now Asiatic cholera had shown a heightened tendency to spread and migrate . . . in the middle of this May in Venice the frightful vibrions were found on one and the same day in the blackish wasted bodies of a cabin boy and a woman who sold greengroceries. The cases were kept secret. But within a week there were ten, twenty, thirty more, and in various sections . . . the food supply had been infected. . . . Cases of recovery were rare. Out of a hundred attacks, eighty were fatal, and in the most horrible manner. For the plague moved with utter savagery. . . ."

Thomas Mann, *Death in Venice*, 1930

WHAT IS THE CHOLERA VACCINE?

The cholera vaccine is composed of whole cholera bacteria that are inactivated with a chemical. The vaccine is not highly effective (the vaccine protects against disease only about 50 percent of the time) and doesn't contain one of the types of bacteria that circulates in India, Bangladesh, and parts of central Asia and eastern Europe.

Two cholera vaccines are made outside the United States: one in Sweden, the other in Switzerland. However, neither of these vaccines is recommended for travelers and both are unavailable in the United States.

In which countries can you catch cholera?

Cholera continues to cause disease in India, Southeast Asia, Africa, the Middle East, southern Europe, the western Pacific Islands (Oceania), South America, and some states of the former Soviet Union (including Ukraine, Azerbaijan, and Armenia). In 1997, about 150,000 cases from sixty-five countries were reported to the World Health Organization.

How can I avoid catching cholera?

Travelers using standard tourist accommodations are at virtually no risk of disease.

However, because the bacterium is spread in water and food (primarily shellfish), the best way to avoid cholera is to make sure that nonbottled water is boiled and that shellfish are adequately cooked.

CHOLERA VACCINE:
SUMMARY AND CONCLUSIONS

Cholera is a common cause of severe diarrhea and death in a number of developing countries. However, travelers using standard tourist accommodations are at virtually no risk of disease. The cholera vaccine is not recommended by the World Health Organization, nor is it required for entry by any country. The cholera vaccine is not available in the United States.

TYPHOID
VACCINE

Tom and Elizabeth are planning a trip to Mexico. They have heard that typhoid fever is common in Mexico and wonder whether there is a vaccine to prevent it.

Typhoid is a disease caused by a bacterium, *Salmonella typhi.* The bacterium causes fever, stomach pain, rash, and in some cases shock and death (called typhoid fever). It is estimated that every year 33 million cases of typhoid fever and 500,000 deaths occur worldwide. The disease primarily occurs in Mexico and the developing countries of South America, Southeast Asia, and Africa.

The typhoid vaccine is not required for international travel, but it is recommended to travelers (under certain circumstances) in areas where the disease is prevalent.

There are two typhoid vaccines available in the United States. Their use depends on the age of the child.

- *Two to six years of age:* One shot of the purified "polysaccharide" vaccine.

- *Six years old or older:* One capsule by mouth of the "Ty21a" vaccine given every other day, for a total of four capsules.

The typhoid vaccine is not recommended for children under two years of age.

Recommendation by the American Academy of Pediatrics and the CDC

The typhoid vaccine is not required for international travel. The vaccine is recommended for anyone traveling to areas of high risk, such as *small towns and rural areas, or who is unlikely to live and eat in standard tourist accommodations*. In addition, the vaccine is recommended for anyone staying for more than six weeks in areas where typhoid is common.

WHAT IS TYPHOID?

Typhoid is a disease caused by a bacterium. The bacterium initially infects the intestines and causes fever, stomach pain, rash, and occasionally shock and death.

"Typhoid Mary"

Mary Mallon ("Typhoid Mary") was infected with typhoid bacteria in the early 1900s while living in New York. Although Mary never had any symptoms, she was contagious to others.

Unfortunately, Mary was a cook who refused to give up her occupation even after many warnings by the health department. She contaminated the food of probably hundreds of people, at least three of whom died of typhoid.

Mary spent the last fifteen years of her life quarantined in a New York City hospital and died in 1930.

WHAT IS THE TYPHOID VACCINE?

There are two typhoid vaccines. The choice of vaccines depends on the age of the child.

- The *oral* vaccine (Ty21a) is a weakened form of the live bacteria.

- The *polysaccharide* vaccine is made of the sugar that coats the bacteria in the same way that the meningococcal vaccine is made.

Both vaccines are between 50 and 80 percent effective at preventing typhoid.

Is the typhoid vaccine safe?

Less than 5 percent of those who receive either the oral typhoid vaccine or the shot will have headache and fever. About 7 percent of those who receive the typhoid shot will have redness and pain where the shot was given.

In which countries can you catch typhoid?

Typhoid is a cause of disease and death primarily in Mexico and in developing countries in Southeast Asia (including India and Pakistan), South America, and Africa.

How can I avoid catching typhoid?

Typhoid is a disease of humans only and is transmitted through the feces. In developing countries, where sewage systems are poor, the disease is transmitted in contaminated water or food. Travelers should drink only bottled water and avoid ice, peeled fruit, undercooked meat, shellfish, salads, or food from street vendors.

The risk of disease is small if travel is limited to tourist accommodations.

Who should get the typhoid vaccine?

Anyone traveling to Mexico, Southeast Asia, South America, and Africa who is likely to enter small towns and rural areas, is staying for more than six weeks, or is unlikely to live and eat in tourist accommodations.

TYPHOID VACCINE:
SUMMARY AND CONCLUSIONS

Typhoid is a bacterium that causes fever, stomach pain, rash, and occasionally shock and death. More than 33 million cases and 500,000 deaths occur each year in the world. The disease is prevalent in developing countries in Asia, South America, and Latin America.

The typhoid vaccines used today are safe and fairly effective. However, because careful travelers are at low risk of catching the disease, the vaccine is recommended only for those who are likely to be exposed to contaminated food or water, those staying for long periods of time, or those staying in rural areas or small towns.

YELLOW FEVER VACCINE

Mary and Liza are planning a trip to Peru and have heard from friends that you can catch yellow fever in South America. They are reassured that the yellow fever vaccine is not required for entry.

If the yellow fever vaccine is not required for entry to Peru, does this also mean that it wouldn't be useful?

Yellow fever is one of the main causes of hepatitis (inflammation of the liver) and hemorrhage (a bleeding disorder) in parts of Africa and South America. Every year throughout the world there are about 200,000 cases of yellow fever, causing as many as 40,000 deaths. Several countries either require or recommend the yellow fever vaccine prior to entry.

WHAT IS YELLOW FEVER?

Yellow fever is a virus that causes inflammation of the liver (hepatitis) as well as severe bleeding problems (hemorrhage). Children usually have fever, chills, muscle pains, headache, and a yellowing of the skin (jaundice). Up to 20 percent of patients with jaundice will die from the disease.

> ### Recommendation by the American Academy of Pediatrics and the CDC
>
> The yellow fever vaccine is either required or recommended for travel to several countries in Africa and South America. It is given as a single shot to children over nine months of age and adults.

WHAT IS THE YELLOW FEVER VACCINE?

The yellow fever vaccine is made in chicken eggs, using a live, weakened form of the virus.

Is the yellow fever vaccine safe?

Side effects from the yellow fever vaccine are rare. About 5 percent of children who receive the vaccine will develop muscle pains and low-grade fever. The yellow fever vaccine should not be given to pregnant women or those with a suppressed immune system caused by leukemia, lymphoma, other cancers, or AIDS. Infants under four months of age should not receive the vaccine because of the increased risk of severe side effects (specifically encephalitis, or inflammation of the brain). In addition, because the yellow fever vaccine is made in eggs, children with egg allergies should not get the vaccine.

In which countries can you catch yellow fever?

Yellow fever is found primarily in Africa and South America. The countries that require a certificate of vaccination for entry from the United States include Benin, Burkina Faso, Cameroon, Central African Republic, Congo, Ivory Coast, French Guiana, Gabon, Ghana, Liberia, Mali, Mauritania, Niger, Rwanda, Senegal, São Tomé, Principe, and Togo.

Countries in South America where yellow fever is prevalent include Brazil, Bolivia, Peru, Equador, Colombia, Panama, Venezuela, Guyana, Suriname, and French Guiana.

How can I avoid catching yellow fever?

Yellow fever is transmitted to children and adults by the bite of a mosquito. The disease is rarely transmitted in urban areas.

Travelers can avoid mosquito bites by staying in air-conditioned or well-screened quarters and wearing long-sleeved shirts and pants. Insect repellents containing DEET should be used only on exposed skin, and repellents containing permethrin should be applied to clothing.

Mosquitoes are most active at sunset and dusk. Therefore, parents should choose indoor or protected activities for their children during these times of the day.

Who should get the yellow fever vaccine?

The yellow fever vaccine is required by the countries listed on page 161 and recommended for travel outside urban areas in countries where the disease is prevalent. A single dose of vaccine provides protection against yellow fever for at least ten years and possibly a lifetime.

Although the vaccine is recommended only for children over nine months of age, children under nine months of age traveling to the countries listed on the previous page may benefit from it if maximal protection against mosquito bites cannot be assured. The yellow fever vaccine should never be given to infants under four months of age.

YELLOW FEVER VACCINE: SUMMARY AND CONCLUSIONS

Every year throughout the world there are about 200,000 cases of yellow fever. The disease is primarily prevalent in certain countries in Africa and South America. Although a certificate of yellow fever vaccination is required for entry into some countries, administration of the vaccine prior to travel to several other countries is also of benefit.

JAPANESE ENCEPHALITIS VIRUS VACCINE

James is being transferred by his company to Japan. He and his family plan to live in Japan for two years before coming back to the United States.

Are there any vaccines specific for travel to the Far East?

Japanese encephalitis virus (JEV) is an occasional cause of outbreaks of encephalitis (inflammation of the brain) primarily in the Far East. Every year about 50,000 cases of JEV occur in the world. Of the children infected with this virus, one in four will die, and half of those who survive will be left with permanent brain damage.

The JEV vaccine is not required for international travel, but it is recommended for travel to certain areas dependent on the length of stay, specific regions visited, and activities planned during travel.

> ## Recommendations by the American Academy of Pediatrics and the CDC
>
> The Japanese encephalitis vaccine is recommended for people traveling to areas where the virus is prevalent and whose length of stay or specific regions of travel (specifically, rural or farming areas) put them at high risk. The vaccine should be given to children at least one year of age and adults as a series of three shots. The last two shots are given seven and thirty days after the first shot.

What Is JEV?

JEV is a virus that causes inflammation of the brain (encephalitis). Afflicted children usually have fever, headache, neck stiffness, nausea, and vomiting. Some children (about 25 percent) will progress to coma and death. Of those who survive, about 50 percent will have seizures and permanent brain damage.

What Is the JEV Vaccine?

The JEV vaccine is made from a virus originally isolated in 1935. The virus is grown in cells from mouse brains, and the vaccine is made by purifying the virus and killing it with formaldehyde.

Is the JEV vaccine safe?

About 20 percent of children given the JEV vaccine will have fever or pain where the shot is given. About 10 percent will have fever, headache, malaise, rash, chills, dizziness, muscle pain, nausea, vomiting, or abdominal pain. About 0.5 percent of vaccinees will have a severe allergic reaction to the JEV vaccine (hives, difficulty breathing).

Because the virus is grown in mouse brains, there has always been concern that the virus may cause side effects in the nervous system. However, this has not been the case.

In which countries can you catch JEV?

JEV is found primarily in Australia, Bangladesh, Brunei, Burma, Cambodia, Hong Kong, India, Indonesia, Japan, Korea, Laos, Malaysia, Nepal, the People's Republic of China, Pakistan, Papua New Guinea, the Philippines, Russia, Singapore, Sri Lanka, Taiwan, Thailand, and Vietnam.

How can I avoid catching JEV?

JEV is transmitted by the bite of a mosquito. The disease is usually transmitted in the summer and early fall (in temperate climates), when mosquitoes are most likely to feed. Mosquitoes usually feed at night, between dusk and dawn.

Travelers can avoid JEV by staying in screened or air-conditioned rooms at dusk and at night. If that is not possible, they should use mosquito netting over beds, as well as insect repellent and protective clothing.

Who should get the JEV vaccine?

The JEV vaccine is not required for international travel, but it is recommended in certain situations.

Travelers to countries listed above who are staying in urban areas or are staying for less than thirty days are at very low risk of catching JEV and are not recommended to receive the vaccine. In contrast, travelers to those countries who will be (1) staying in rural or farm areas, (2) staying for more than thirty days, or (3) planning activities such as biking, camping, or other unprotected outdoor activities should consider getting the vaccine.

Travelers should call either local travel clinics or the Centers for Disease Control and Prevention in Atlanta (1-877-394-8747) to determine in which seasons JEV is prevalent in their destinations.

Japanese Encephalitis Vaccine: Summary and Conclusions

Every year about 50,000 people in the world are infected with Japanese encephalitis virus. Many either die or are left with permanent brain damage from this infection. In several countries in the Far East, the virus either circulates all the time or occurs in epidemics. For travelers to these countries, the vaccine is not required when travel will be confined to urban areas and will be for less than thirty days. However, if travel will include rural areas or last for longer than thirty days, Japanese encephalitis vaccine should be considered. The best way to make this decision is to call the CDC at 1-877-394-8747 and determine the months in which the virus is prevalent in your area of travel.

PART FIVE

VACCINES FOR
THE FUTURE

ROTAVIRUS VACCINE ("THE VOMITING/ DIARRHEA VACCINE")

The rotavirus vaccine ("Rotashield") was licensed by the Food and Drug Administration on August 31, 1998, and recommended by the Centers for Disease Control and Prevention (CDC) for all children in the United States. The vaccine was given by mouth as a series of three doses at two months, four months, and six months of age. However, in October 1999, after approximately 1 million children had been immunized with the rotavirus vaccine, the CDC withdrew its recommendation when it found that the rotavirus vaccine was a rare cause of an intestinal problem called "intussusception." Approximately one of every 10,000 children who got the rotavirus vaccine developed intussusception. Intussusception occurs when a part of the intestine folds in on itself and causes intestinal blockage, pain, cramping, and blood in the stools. The disease is serious, causing children to be admitted to the hospital. The intestinal blockage is treated with either a barium enema or surgery.

Because rotavirus infects all children in the United States by three years of age, a discontinuation of the "rotavirus vaccine program" meant a continuation of the "rotavirus disease program." Every year in the United States rotavirus infections cause about 500,000 children to visit their doctor, 160,000 to visit the emergency room, 50,000 to be hospitalized, and forty to die. Pharmaceutical companies are now charged with making a safer rotavirus vaccine as quickly and efficiently as possible. In this chapter we discuss the impact of rotavirus infections as well as future rotavirus vaccines.

Most parents are aware that during the winter months their young children may have a bout with diarrhea. What many parents don't know is that the most common cause of fever, vomiting, and diarrhea in children under three years of age has a name: rotavirus.

Every winter in the United States, rotavirus will infect about 2 million infants and young children. Because the virus causes both fever and vomiting (in addition to diarrhea), it is often difficult to give children all the fluids they need. The result is that about 50,000 children will be admitted to the hospital every year in the United States with dehydration (water loss) caused by rotavirus. *That means that one out of every seventy-five children born in this country will be hospitalized with rotavirus infection.*

What Is Rotavirus?

Rotavirus is a virus that infects the intestines. The infection causes fever, vomiting, and diarrhea lasting for about one week. Those most severely infected are between six months and two years of age.

Rotavirus infections are so common that *every* child in the United States will be infected at least once by three years of age. Many children are infected two or three times within the first few years of life.

How Was the First Rotavirus Vaccine Made?

The strategy used to make the first rotavirus vaccine was different from that for any other vaccine. The vaccine was a combination of strains of rotavirus that caused disease in children and a strain of rotavirus that infected monkeys.

Practically every mammal on earth is infected by its own unique rotavirus strains. So rotavirus not only infects children, it also infects the young of many other species. However, rotavirus that infects one species isn't very efficient at infecting the young of another. For example, although cow (or bovine) rotavirus can cause severe diarrhea in calves, it doesn't cause diarrhea in children.

The first rotavirus vaccine was made by combining monkey rotavirus with a human rotavirus (called a "combination" or "reassortant" virus). The human-monkey reassortant viruses had two important features. The human part of the reassortant viruses caused immunity that protected children against severe disease. The monkey part of the reassortant viruses weakened the viruses so that children didn't vomit or get diarrhea from the vaccine.

Was the first rotavirus vaccine safe?

The CDC and the American Academy of Pediatrics withdrew their recommendations to use the first rotavirus vaccine when it was found to be a rare cause of intussusception in children.

Intussusception occurs when the intestine (which is a long, narrow tube) folds into itself. When this happens, blood supply to the intestine is cut off, and the result is intestinal blockage, pain, cramping, and blood in the stools. Intussusception is a medical emergency and requires children to be admitted to the hospital.

The rotavirus vaccine was given to about 1 million children in the United States between 1998 and 1999. About one of every 10,000 children who were given the vaccine got intussusception (a total of about 100 children) and one child died because of the vaccine. The CDC and the AAP felt that this risk from the first rotavirus vaccine was simply too great and preferred to wait for a rotavirus vaccine that was safer.

But what about children who didn't get the rotavirus vaccine? If you look at 1 million children who didn't get the vaccine, about 16,000 were hospitalized with water loss (or dehydration) and about five to ten died from dehydration caused by rotavirus. So, many more children were hospitalized and killed by rotavirus infection than were hospitalized and killed by the rotavirus vaccine. The choice not to give the vaccine was not a risk-free choice—it was simply a choice to take a different risk.

Can we expect that future rotavirus vaccines would be safer?

Two other rotavirus vaccines are currently being developed. Neither of these two vaccines uses the monkey rotavirus strain contained in the first rotavirus vaccine. One vaccine contains a combination of a cow (or bovine) rotavirus and human rotavirus. This bovine-human rotavirus vaccine does not appear to cause any side effects in preliminary trials. Another rotavirus vaccine strategy uses a weakened form of human rotavirus. In both cases, about 60,000 children may need to be immunized in clinical trials before the vaccine is made available. This should help us to determine whether either of these vaccines causes intussusception before they are licensed for use in children.

Why should we prevent a disease as mild as diarrhea?

The disease caused by rotavirus is usually not mild.

The reason that rotavirus infections are so severe is that most infected children have both vomiting and fever in addition to the diarrhea. This means that not only do children lose fluids because of diarrhea, but it is also difficult to replace the fluids lost because of the vomiting and high fever. Sometimes rotavirus infections are so severe that children become dehydrated within one day of the beginning of symptoms.

ROTAVIRUS VACCINE: SUMMARY AND CONCLUSIONS

Because the first rotavirus vaccine was withdrawn for use, rotavirus infections remain an important cause of fever, vomiting, diarrhea, hospitalizations, and occasionally death in this country. It is now incumbent upon us to make a safer rotavirus vaccine as quickly and efficiently as possible.

CHAPTER 27

LYME DISEASE VACCINE

In 1998, a vaccine to prevent Lyme disease was licensed by the Food and Drug Administration and recommended for use. In 2002, the Lyme vaccine was discontinued by the manufacturer. In this chapter we discuss how the Lyme vaccine was made, how it worked, whether it was safe, and why it was discontinued.

Lyme disease is caused by a bacterium called *Borrelia burgdorferi* that is transmitted by the bite of a tick. The disease affects the joints, skin, nervous system, and heart and, if left untreated, can cause permanent damage to those tissues. About 15,000 people each year develop Lyme disease in the United States.

WHAT IS LYME DISEASE?

Lyme disease was first recognized in 1975 when several children from Lyme, Connecticut, were initially believed to have a form of childhood arthritis (inflammation of the joints). The disease was called Lyme arthritis until it became clear that more than just the joints were involved.

Lyme disease is caused by a bacterium that is transmitted by the bite of a tick. The name of the bacterium is *Borrelia burgdorferi*. Within a few days to a few weeks, the bacteria infect the skin that surrounds the tick bite and cause a red, circular rash, often with a pale center. The rash is accompanied by headache, fever, chills, achiness, and swollen glands.

Within a few weeks to a few months of the tick bite, the bacteria can also damage areas other than the skin. Joints such as the knee often become hot, tender, and swollen. Joint symptoms can recur over a period of several years.

Excruciating headaches and neck pain occur when the bacteria infect the lining of the brain, causing meningitis. In addition, the bacteria can infect the brain itself (causing encephalitis) or individual nerves. For example, some people with Lyme disease are unable to move the muscles on one side of their face (called a facial palsy, or Bell's palsy). This facial palsy is often the only symptom of Lyme disease.

Lyme bacteria can also cause an irregular heart rate, or arrhythmia.

What Was the Lyme Vaccine?

The bacterium that causes Lyme disease is coated by several proteins called outer surface proteins, or Osp. An immune response directed against these proteins appears to protect against disease.

The vaccine consisted of one of the surface proteins (OspA). Adolescents and adults immunized with the Lyme vaccine developed antibodies to the OspA protein. These antibodies protected against Lyme disease in an unusual manner. When an immunized person was bitten by a tick, the OspA antibodies entered the body of the tick while it was taking a blood meal. These antibodies neutralized the Lyme bacteria before it actually entered a person's body!

About 50 percent of people immunized with the Lyme vaccine were protected against Lyme disease after two doses, and about 75 percent were protected after three doses.

Who gets Lyme disease?

Lyme disease has been reported in forty-seven states. However, children and adults are most likely to get Lyme disease if they live in the

Northeast (from Massachusetts to Maryland), the Midwest (Wisconsin and Minnesota), or the West (California and Oregon). Most disease occurs in June and July. In some areas (such as Nantucket, Massachusetts) as many as 10 percent of all residents have been infected with the Lyme bacteria.

People who get Lyme disease are those who engage in activities that result in frequent or prolonged exposure to tick-infested areas. Recreational, property-maintenance, occupational, or leisure activities all may result in sufficient exposure.

Avoiding tick-infested areas—and increasing personal protection by wearing high socks and applying insect repellants containing DEET—can reduce the incidence of tick bites. However, these methods do not provide complete protection against the risk of Lyme disease.

Lyme disease does not infect one particular age group; anyone at any age who is bitten by a tick is at risk.

Was the Lyme vaccine safe?

The Lyme vaccine was given to about 11,000 people before it was licensed for use in the United States, and symptoms were monitored for about twenty months. About 20 percent of people reported soreness at the site of injection; less than 2 percent reported redness and swelling. Muscle aches, fever, and chills (flu-like illness) were reported in less than 3 percent of those immunized.

People who had already been exposed to the Lyme bacteria (meaning people who already had Lyme antibodies in their blood) did not have an increased incidence of adverse effects as compared with those who had not been previously exposed.

Why was the Lyme vaccine discontinued?

The Lyme vaccine was recommended for use in adolescents and adults fifteen to seventy years of age who lived, worked, or played in areas where Lyme disease occurred. The vaccine was given as a series of three shots.

In 1998, when the Lyme vaccine was first licensed, a publication in the journal *Science* caused some concerns. Concerns focused on people with Lyme disease and long-term swelling and pain in the joints (arthritis). The study found that people with a certain genetic background with recurrent arthritis caused by the Lyme bacteria might be reacting to a component of the bacteria that is similar to a component of their bodies. In other words, in response to the Lyme bacteria, people made antibodies to the various components of the bacteria, but inadvertently also made antibodies to themselves (called autoimmunity). The reason that this finding raised concerns about the Lyme vaccine was that the component of the bacteria to which these patients were responding was also a component of the vaccine.

However, subsequent studies showed that people who received the vaccine were not at greater risk of arthritis than people who did not receive the vaccine. This finding is consistent with the fact that vaccination is very different from natural infection. Natural infection can cause mild destruction of the joints and cause a release of the protein that is similar to the Lyme protein contained in the bacteria. However, vaccination with part of the Lyme bacteria doesn't cause destruction of the joint and so doesn't cause the release of the protein. If the protein isn't released, then the immune system doesn't react to it and cause autoimmunity.

Unfortunately, some people were not reassured by the data showing no increase in arthritis following the use of the Lyme vaccine. Controversy surrounding the safety of the Lyme vaccine limited its use and ultimately caused the manufacturer to discontinue the vaccine. The sad part of this story is that every year in the United States about 15,000 people will suffer from Lyme disease and some will go on to develop complications of the joints, heart, and nervous system. A technology that safely and effectively prevents this suffering is now no longer available.

Lyme Disease and Bites

Lyme disease is not only the most common tick-transmitted disease in the United States, but the most common insect-transmitted disease (including diseases spread by flies, mosquitoes, and fleas).

I thought that antibiotics cured Lyme disease. Why was it necessary to prevent Lyme disease with a vaccine?

Several antibiotics can be used to treat Lyme disease effectively. If someone is bitten by a tick and develops early symptoms of Lyme disease, prompt recognition of the disease and appropriate treatment with antibiotics usually means that the infection will be mild.

Unfortunately, Lyme disease is sometimes not diagnosed in the early stages of infection and appropriate antibiotics are not prescribed. When this happens, the infection can spread to the joints and, in rare instances, to the nervous system or heart. Although appropriate antibiotics can cure Lyme disease even in the late stages, the best solution to the dilemma would be to have an effective vaccine. Also, a few people diagnosed early and treated correctly for Lyme disease still go on to develop joint, nervous system, or heart problems.

LYME VACCINE: SUMMARY AND CONCLUSIONS

Lyme disease can damage the joints, nervous system, and heart. Prompt recognition and treatment of this disease is sometimes necessary to avoid the possibility of permanent damage.

Unfortunately, early infection with Lyme disease may be difficult to recognize. The best way to avoid the damage caused by the disease is to prevent it with a vaccine. Unfortunately, although there was no evidence that the Lyme vaccine was harmful, controversy surrounding the safety of the vaccine limited its use. In 2002, the Lyme vaccine was discontinued by the manufacturer.

COMBINATION VACCINES

Trent is two months old. His mother takes him to the pediatrician and finds out that he needs four vaccines, all of which are given as shots (DTaP, Hib, Hep B, and IPV). She asks the doctor whether there is some way he can get these vaccines without getting so many shots.

Eleven vaccines are recommended for routine use in all children. Of those, six are given in combination. The diphtheria, tetanus, and pertussis vaccines are combined to make DTaP; and the measles, mumps, and rubella vaccines are combined to make MMR. However, the recent addition of new vaccines such as Hib, varicella, hepatitis B, pneumococcus, and the inactivated polio vaccine (IPV) have dramatically increased the number of shots that a child receives in the first year of life. It is now possible for a child to receive as many as five shots in a single visit (DTaP, IPV, Hib, pneumococcus, and hepatitis B). This can be distressing to both the child and the parent.

Sometimes parents will ask their doctors whether they can draw up each of the different vaccines into a single syringe and give it to their child as a single shot. Unfortunately, it's not that easy. Sometimes either the stabilizer or buffer for one vaccine (and even the vaccine itself) will interfere with the capacity of another vaccine to induce immunity.

The good news is that help is on the way. Several companies are now working together to combine vaccines. The following combinations are either recently licensed or in progress:

- A combination of hepatitis B and Hib was licensed in October of 1996 and became available in early 1997.

- Vaccines that include DTaP, IPV, Hep B, or Hib should be available soon.

- A combination of measles, mumps, rubella, and varicella is currently being tested in clinical trials and should be available soon.

Use of these combination vaccines will clearly reduce the number of shots required in the first year of life.

CHAPTER 29

RESPIRATORY SYNCYTIAL VIRUS VACCINE ("THE VIRAL PNEUMONIA VACCINE")

Jenny is eighteen months old. One day she developed a high fever and difficulty breathing. She was having so much trouble breathing that it was hard for her to hold down fluids. At the doctor's office, Jenny's mother was told that Jenny was wheezing. The results of the chest X-ray showed that Jenny had pneumonia. The doctor told Jenny's mother that Jenny would need to go to the hospital to receive oxygen therapy and intravenous fluids.

Could anything have been done to prevent this?

Respiratory syncytial virus, or RSV, is the most common cause of severe lung disease in young children. The first time a child is infected with RSV, he or she usually develops pneumonia or bronchiolitis (inflammation of the small breathing tubes, causing wheezing). Virtually every child will be infected by two years of age.

Every year about 90,000 children are hospitalized and 5,000 die from infections caused by RSV. That means that about one out of every forty children born in this country will be hospitalized with RSV disease.

Although recent clinical trials have shown some promise, it is unlikely that an RSV vaccine will be available soon.

WHAT IS RESPIRATORY SYNCYTIAL VIRUS?

An infection with RSV begins with fever and a runny nose that lasts about three days. Children then develop difficulty breathing, rapid breathing, and a deepening cough. First-time infections with RSV usually occur by two years of age and are quite severe. More than 50 percent of children infected with the virus for the first time will develop either pneumonia or bronchiolitis (inflammation of the small breathing tubes of the lung). RSV also can cause croup (inflammation of the vocal cords and windpipe). Many children infected with RSV for the first time need to be hospitalized.

Children usually catch RSV from other children who are coughing or sneezing. The disease is highly contagious.

RSV and Ear Infections

Respiratory syncytial virus commonly causes ear infections. However, because RSV is a virus, it is not killed by antibiotics. Therefore, many children are given antibiotics unnecessarily for ear infections caused by RSV.

Why is it important to prevent RSV?

No drug cures RSV infection. Therefore, the only way to avoid the damage caused by RSV will be to develop a successful vaccine.

Other than waiting for a vaccine, is there anything I can do to prevent RSV in my children?

There is a medicine to prevent RSV infection called Synagis, which is recommended for use by the American Academy of Pediatrics (AAP). Synagis contains antibodies directed against RSV. Because children who were born prematurely (less than 32 weeks' gestation) and those who have lung disease from prematurity are at high risk of severe and occasionally fatal RSV infections, the AAP now recommends that Synagis be considered for use in these children. The medication is given as a shot once a month for five months prior to and during the winter season (when RSV is most likely to occur).

Although Synagis is of some value in preventing RSV infections, it is of no value in treating infections.

When can we expect to have an RSV vaccine?

There are no immediate prospects for an RSV vaccine.

Many approaches to develop a vaccine have been tried, using live, weakened virus, killed virus, and purified viral proteins (see Chapter 3). Recent trials of an RSV vaccine in children with cystic fibrosis have shown some promise. Unfortunately, no vaccines have been proven clearly effective, and it is unlikely that one will be available soon.

RSV Vaccine:
Summary and Conclusions

RSV causes severe pneumonia and wheezing in infants and young children. Virtually every child will be infected with RSV within the first few years of life, and as many as one out of every 40 children born in this country will be hospitalized because of this infection. Unfortunately, it is unlikely that an RSV vaccine for use in all children will be available soon.

CHAPTER 30

AIDS VACCINE

Elizabeth is twenty-five years old. She contracted HIV, the virus that causes AIDS, from a blood transfusion when she was in the hospital twenty years ago. She is interested in getting married and wonders whether a vaccine could be given to her future husband to eliminate his risk of getting AIDS.

Will there soon be a vaccine to prevent AIDS?

AIDS stands for *A*cquired *I*mmunodeficiency *S*yndrome. This disease is caused by the human immunodeficiency virus, or HIV. About 570,000 people in the United States have AIDS, and at least 6,000 of them are children.

Despite the enormous amount of time and money spent on understanding this disease, there are no immediate prospects for a vaccine. In this chapter we discuss who gets AIDS, what the symptoms are, and why it has been so hard to develop an effective AIDS vaccine.

WHAT IS AIDS?

AIDS was first described in 1980. At that time, physicians in Los Angeles, New York, and San Francisco noticed that some young homosexual men either were infected by unusual microorganisms or had developed unusual cancers. In addition, the immune systems of these men were deficient: white blood cells (called lymphocytes) in the blood of these patients were either absent or few in number. Lymphocytes are important in helping the body fight infections.

Because these immunologic deficiencies were occurring in previously healthy men, the disease was thought to have been recently acquired (as distinct from inherited or congenital). The syndrome was, therefore, called acquired immunodeficiency syndrome, or AIDS.

In 1983, the disease was found to be caused by a virus that was later called human immunodeficiency virus, or HIV. The discovery of the virus that caused AIDS allowed scientists to develop a blood test. This blood test enabled doctors to tell whether someone was infected with HIV and whether blood that was used in transfusions was contaminated with the virus.

AIDS Is Spreading Across the World

AIDS was initially seen in North America, western Europe, and sub-Saharan Africa. Now every continent on earth has people infected with HIV.

About 30 million people (including 10 million children) are infected with HIV. In some parts of Africa, as many as 40 percent of young women are infected with HIV.

How can you tell whether someone has AIDS?

Some people who are infected with HIV initially don't have any symptoms. Others have fever, headache, swollen glands, and a sore throat that lasts for one or two weeks. These people are said to be HIV-infected.

About half of the people infected with HIV will develop more severe symptoms within ten years. Once they have developed severe symptoms, they are said to have AIDS. The symptoms that indicate that a patient may have AIDS are pneumonia caused by an unusual fungus (called *Pneumocystis carinii*), infection of the esophagus caused by a fungus (*Candida albicans*), or progressive loss of weight and energy (known as "wasting" syndrome).

Children who have AIDS get two additional diseases when they first develop severe symptoms. They might develop an unusual pneumonia of uncertain cause, as well as different kinds of recurrent bacterial infections.

How do children and adults get AIDS?

Children usually get AIDS by coming in contact with HIV-infected blood. Babies can become infected either while still in the womb or while passing through the birth canal of a mother with HIV. Also, children might have received blood transfusions from people who were infected with HIV.

Adults usually get AIDS by having sexual contact (either homosexual or heterosexual) with people who are infected with HIV. They can also get AIDS by receiving a blood transfusion from or sharing a syringe with someone who was infected with HIV.

The availability of a blood test for AIDS has virtually eliminated transfused blood as a source of HIV in the United States.

Why is it important to prevent AIDS?

Several drugs are available that help stop the growth of HIV in the body. These drugs both prolong the time from infection with HIV to development of AIDS and prolong the life of people who have AIDS after symptoms develop.

Unfortunately, because there is presently no cure for AIDS, the best hope to eliminate the disease will be to prevent it with an effective vaccine.

When will an AIDS vaccine be available?

Despite intensive worldwide efforts to understand the structure of HIV, how it causes disease, and how the body fights to prevent the disease, an effective vaccine is not at hand.

One of the reasons that it has been so hard to make an effective HIV vaccine is that the HIV strain that infects one person may be different from the strain that infects another. Researchers have tried to identify parts of the virus that are similar among many different strains and determine whether they would be suitable for a vaccine.

It is unlikely that there will be an effective HIV vaccine soon.

AIDS Vaccine:
Summary and Conclusions

About 570,000 people, including about 6,000 children, in the United States have AIDS. The disease is often fatal. Although the National Institutes of Health, as well as a number of pharmaceutical companies, have devoted considerable efforts to the development of an AIDS vaccine, there are no immediate prospects. It is unlikely that there will be a vaccine available to prevent AIDS soon.

PART SIX

VACCINES FOR BIOTERRORIST AGENTS AND OTHER CONSIDERATIONS

CHAPTER 31

SMALLPOX VACCINE

Elizabeth is twenty-five years old. She knows that smallpox infections no longer occur anywhere in the world, but is afraid that the events of September 11, 2001, make smallpox a potential agent for bioterrorist attacks. She wonders whether a smallpox vaccine is still made and, if so, whether she should get it.

WHAT IS SMALLPOX?

Smallpox is a virus. Symptoms of smallpox infection begin with high fever, malaise, and backache followed by the development of a rash. The rash begins in the lining of the mouth and throat as well as on the face and forearms before spreading to the trunk and legs. The rash starts with red bumps that are flat to the skin, but progresses to raised bumps, blisters, and finally scabs. The time from the beginning of the rash to the formation of scabs is about two weeks. The rash of smallpox is deeply embedded in the skin. Residual, lifelong pockmarks on the skin often occur following resolution of the illness.

About 30 percent of people infected with smallpox die from the disease.

How do you catch smallpox?

Smallpox is very contagious and is spread from one person to another by tiny droplets from the mouth and throat. The virus is spread by coughing, sneezing, or talking. Contact with an infected person must be fairly close (within about six feet) in order for it to be spread.

Smallpox is different from chickenpox in how it is spread. Whereas chickenpox virus (varicella) can be spread before the rash occurs, smallpox is spread only after the rash has occurred. The virus that is spread from one person to another is contained in the blisters that are located in the mouth and throat. Usually it takes about twelve days from the time one is exposed to the virus to the beginning of symptoms.

The Face of Smallpox

Five European monarchs died from smallpox. When Cortez brought smallpox from Europe to the Western Hemisphere, about 4 million Aztecs died from the disease. In the early part of the eighteenth century, Boston, at that time a city of 10,000 people, suffered an epidemic of smallpox; 5,000 people were infected and 800 died. Indeed, smallpox has probably killed more people in the history of the world than all other infectious diseases combined! About 300 million people have died from smallpox.

WHAT IS THE SMALLPOX VACCINE?

The smallpox vaccine is made using a poxvirus that infects cows (cowpox, or vaccinia). Cowpox causes disease in cows, but it rarely causes disease in humans. Because cowpox and human smallpox are similar, infection with cowpox can protect humans against smallpox.

The person who first used cowpox to protect against smallpox was Edward Jenner, in 1796. Jenner was a family physician who lived in southern England. He noticed that every few years, when smallpox would sweep across the English countryside, women who milked cows (milkmaids) were spared the infection. He reasoned that these women were getting infected during milking when they came in contact with blisters on the udders of cows that had cowpox. This infection protected the milkmaids from infection with smallpox. So, Jenner took fluid from the blisters of cows and injected it into humans to see if that fluid protected them against smallpox. It worked.

By 1977, smallpox, the most feared and devastating of all infectious diseases, was eliminated from the face of the earth. The last case of natural smallpox occurred in Somalia.

However, due to fears that smallpox virus might be used as a biologic agent of terror, the United States recently began to make the smallpox vaccine again. About 300 million doses of smallpox will be available by early 2003.

How is the smallpox vaccine administered?

The smallpox vaccine is administered in a unique manner. A drop of cowpox is placed on the upper arm. The drop is then inoculated into the skin using a two-pronged, stainless steel needle. The needle is used to puncture the skin about thirty times. The vaccination often causes a residual, lifelong scar.

Does the smallpox vaccine have side effects?

The smallpox vaccine initially causes a red, raised bump at the site of inoculation that progresses to a blister and eventually a scab. The scab then separates from the skin about two weeks after inoculation.

Mild side effects from the vaccine include fever and swelling of the lymph node in the armpit near the site of inoculation. About 70 percent of people given the vaccine will have a fever greater than 100°C. The fever usually begins about four days after inoculation.

Severe side effects following administration of the smallpox vaccine do occur, but are relatively uncommon:

- About five of every 10,000 people given the vaccine will inadvertently transfer the virus from the site of inoculation to another site (usually the eyelid, face, nose, mouth, genitals, or rectum). Inadvertent inoculation can cause swelling, tenderness, and rash at the site of transfer.

- About two of every 10,000 people given the vaccine will develop a generalized rash that spreads to the body. The generalized rash occurs more commonly in people with eczema.

- About one of every 100,000 people who get the smallpox vaccine will develop an infection of their brain called encephalitis.

- About one of every 1,000,000 people given the smallpox vaccine will develop a severe progressive form of the disease that is often fatal. These people usually have severe immunologic deficits prior to receipt of the vaccine.

Who should get the smallpox vaccine?

The smallpox vaccine was at one time given routinely to all children in the United States at about one year of age. By the 1960s, the risk of smallpox in the United States was dramatically reduced. Therefore, because the risks of the vaccine outweighed its benefits, routine administration of the smallpox vaccine to infants in the United States was discontinued in 1971. Administration to health-care workers was discontinued in 1976; administration to international travelers was discontinued in 1982; and administration to military personnel was discontinued in 1990.

Smallpox vaccine is no longer recommended for use. However, recent events have necessitated immunizing both local and federal public health clinicians, who would be the first to respond to a potential bioterrorist attack. Currently, the smallpox vaccine is not recommended for routine use.

How long does immunity to smallpox last?

The smallpox vaccine was discontinued for routine use in the United States in the early 1970s. So, most people in this country younger than thirty years of age have never been vaccinated against smallpox. But what about people over thirty? Does immunity to smallpox last thirty years or longer?

The best study to answer this question was performed in England in the early 1900s. An outbreak of smallpox affecting more than 1,000 people occurred in Liverpool between 1902 and 1903. People infected with smallpox were divided into two groups: those who got smallpox vaccine in infancy and those who did not. The fatality rate for thirty- to forty-nine-year-olds was about 4 percent in the vaccinated group and 54 percent in the unvaccinated group. For those older than fifty years of age, the fatality rate was about 6 percent in the vaccinated group and 50 percent in the unvaccinated group.

Therefore, smallpox vaccine protected against disease caused by smallpox, even fifty years after vaccination.

Do the benefits of the smallpox vaccine outweigh its risks?

No. As of this writing, smallpox infections no longer occur in the world. Currently, the risks of the vaccine outweigh its benefits. However, if smallpox infections occurred again in the world, the relationship between vaccine risks and benefits would change dramatically.

ANTHRAX
VACCINE

Kellam is twenty-eight years old. She works in New York City, where a few people have contracted anthrax. She wonders whether she would benefit from getting the anthrax vaccine.

WHAT IS ANTHRAX?

The disease anthrax is caused by the bacterium *Bacillus anthracis*. Spores of this bacterium live in the soil and are eaten by grazing livestock. People get anthrax when they come in contact with infected animals. Therefore, slaughterhouse workers are most likely to get anthrax.

How do you catch anthrax?

Most cases of anthrax occur when bacteria enter the skin through a cut or abrasion (cutaneous [or skin] anthrax) in people who are handling contaminated meat, wool, hides, leather, or hair products from infected animals. About one to seven days after exposure, symptoms of anthrax begin as a small red area on the skin that progresses to a blackened,

194

painless ulcer. Soon lymph glands begin to swell and the patient may have fever, tiredness, and headache. If untreated, about 20 percent of those infected will develop difficulty breathing and a bloodstream infection that causes death. If treated with antibiotics, less than 1 percent of infected persons will die.

Very rarely, people will inhale enough spores to cause disease (called inhalational anthrax). Humans have to breathe in about 8,000 to 50,000 spores to get the inhalational form of anthrax. Symptoms usually begin about nine to ten days after inhalation and include sore throat, mild fever, and muscle aches. Symptoms then progress to severe difficulty in breathing and shock. If untreated, inhalational anthrax is often fatal. Anthrax can also infect the lining of the brain and spinal cord, causing meningitis.

How could anthrax be used as a biological weapon?

Theoretically, anthrax spores distributed in the air could be used to kill large numbers of people (inhalational anthrax). However, for several reasons, anthrax has limitations as a biological weapon. First, it is not easy to grow the virulent form of the bacteria in culture so that it makes spores. The temperature has to be hot enough to create spores but not too hot to kill the spores. Second, one would need to generate pounds of spores to cause the deaths of many people. Third, spores must be present in the air in large quantities for several hours to cause disease. Therefore, spores would have to be distributed through a nozzle that is just the right size. If the nozzle is too large, spores will clump together and settle quickly to the ground. Once on the ground, the spores are not likely to cause disease. Fourth, wind currents could dramatically affect the distribution of spores. If spores were distributed over a large city or sporting event, wind currents would probably disperse spores and reduce their concentration in the air. Fifth, anthrax is not contagious. People don't spread the disease to other people. Sixth, anthrax can be treated with antibiotics such as penicillin, doxycycline, and ciprofloxacin.

As of this writing, anthrax has been distributed only by letters containing relatively small quantities of anthrax spores. This suggests the lack of a capacity or expertise to manufacture large quantities of anthrax and distribute them broadly.

WHAT IS THE ANTHRAX VACCINE?

The anthrax vaccine is made by taking a strain of the bacteria *Bacillus anthracis* and growing it in the laboratory. The bacteria releases several harmful proteins, called toxins, into the surrounding broth. These toxins are responsible for disease in those infected with the anthrax bacteria. The toxins are then inactivated with formaldehyde so that they can no longer cause disease. Anthrax bacteria are filtered out of the vaccine. Thus, the anthrax vaccine is made in a manner similar to the acellular pertussis vaccine (see Chapter 7).

Who should get the anthrax vaccine?

The anthrax vaccine is available in limited supply and usually only for military personnel. The vaccine is given as a series of six shots. After the first shot, the vaccine is given two weeks, four weeks, six months, twelve months, and eighteen months later.

Currently, a vaccine is being developed that can be given as two shots.

Does the anthrax vaccine work?

More than 95 percent of people given three doses of the anthrax vaccine will develop high levels of antibodies against anthrax in their blood. The effectiveness of the anthrax vaccine is not well studied, but one study, published in 1962, had interesting results. Mill workers at high risk of getting anthrax were given either vaccine or no vaccine. The effectiveness of the vaccine was about 92 percent. What was of interest in this study was that, during the study, an outbreak of inhalational anthrax occurred. Inhalational anthrax occurs when large numbers of anthrax spores are released in the air and is analogous to what would happen if anthrax were used as a biological weapon. Five people got anthrax disease after breathing in the anthrax spores—all five of these people had not received the vaccine.

Therefore, the anthrax vaccine appears to be effective in preventing inhalational anthrax.

Does the anthrax vaccine have side effects?

About one of every five people who receive the anthrax vaccine develop mild pain, redness, and swelling at the site where the vaccine was given.

And about one out of every 100 people given the vaccine develop severe pain and swelling. In addition, four of every 7,000 people who get the anthrax vaccine have fever, chills, body aches, or nausea. A severe allergic reaction (called anaphylaxis) that includes difficulty in breathing, hives, or lowered blood pressure can occur but is extremely rare.

Did the anthrax vaccine cause Gulf War Syndrome?

A long-lasting disease that included muscle pain, fatigue, and headaches was associated with deployment of military personnel to the Gulf War. Some people wondered whether the Gulf War syndrome (GWS) was caused by the anthrax vaccine. To determine whether anthrax vaccine caused GWS, a study was performed. Blood was taken from people who complained of symptoms of GWS and from those who did not. The percentage of people who had antibodies to anthrax was not different between the two groups. Therefore, the anthrax vaccine does not appear to be the cause of GWS.

Do antibiotics treat anthrax?

Antibiotics such as penicillin, doxycycline, and ciprofloxacin all have been found to kill the anthrax bacteria and can effectively treat patients with anthrax.

Should I keep antibiotics such as ciprofloxacin (Cipro) in my house in case of a bioterrorist attack?

Antibiotics should *not* be stored in the home for several reasons. First, antibiotics are best used to treat, not to prevent, anthrax infection. Therefore, antibiotics should be used only after an exposure has been known or suspected to have occurred. So far, not very many people have been exposed to anthrax in a country of about 280 million people. The risk of exposure is, therefore, very low. Second, if many people stockpile antibiotics such as ciprofloxacin, available antibiotic supplies will be depleted and lesser quantities will be available for mobilization to an area that might become affected. Third, inappropriate use of antibiotics could potentially cause common strains of other bacteria to become resistant and, therefore, more difficult to treat when they cause infection.

If antibiotics treat anthrax, why do military personnel need a vaccine?

The problem with antibiotics is that they can kill the anthrax bacteria, but they can't kill the anthrax spores. If there were a bioterrorist attack, spores would be released into the air and inhaled. Antibiotics would prevent the development of the disease, but would not necessarily kill all the spores. If someone took antibiotics for several weeks, or even several months, and then stopped taking antibiotics, the spores could become active (germinate) and cause disease. It is unclear exactly how long antibiotics should be given before it is certain that all the inhaled spores inhaled can't germinate, but the best guess is about six weeks.

Also, not all people with anthrax who are treated with antibiotics survive. As with all diseases in medicine, prevention is always better than treatment. For these reasons, the anthrax vaccine is of value.

Do the Benefits of the Anthrax Vaccine Outweigh the Risks?

Anthrax bacteria could be used in an attack against the United States during a conflict or as an agent of terror. If a person inhales anthrax spores and is not treated with antibiotics, it is possible that the spores would cause a fatal infection. Since not all people with anthrax who are treated with antibiotics survive, and because the length of treatment for someone who has inhaled spores is unclear, the anthrax vaccine is of value. The anthrax vaccine has a side effect profile similar to the vaccines routinely recommended for children. The benefits of the anthrax vaccine outweigh the risks for those at highest risk of infection (that is, military personnel).

VACCINES FOR TEENAGERS

Jon is fifteen years old. His mother takes him to the doctor's office for a camp physical and finds out that he needs to get several vaccines. Jon's mother thought that he had already gotten all the vaccines he needed.

Are there vaccines specifically for teenagers?

Because teenagers don't get routine medical checkups, they aren't very good about getting the vaccines they need. Only 5 percent of fifteen- to nineteen-year-olds regularly visit their doctor. Most teenagers (and adults) wrongly assume that the vaccines they got as children were all that they needed for the rest of their lives.

The American Academy of Pediatrics now recommends a routine visit to the doctor for all children eleven to twelve years of age to provide the opportunity to receive four different vaccine preparations: varicella, hepatitis B, measles-mumps-rubella, and tetanus-diphtheria. For incoming college freshmen, the meningococcal vaccine is also of value. In this chapter we discuss why it is important that teenagers get each of these vaccines.

VARICELLA (CHICKENPOX) VACCINE

The varicella vaccine should be given to all teenagers who have not yet had chickenpox. Children who have managed to get to thirteen years of age without getting chickenpox are at high risk of severe disease when they get varicella. This is because older teenagers and adults are more likely to develop pneumonia or encephalitis (inflammation of the brain) and are fifteen times more likely to die from chickenpox than young children. For these reasons, the varicella vaccine was recently recommended for use in *all* children up to eighteen years of age. About 20 percent of adolescents have never had chickenpox.

Recommendation by the American Academy of Pediatrics

A single dose of the varicella vaccine is recommended to be given to all children between eleven and twelve years of age who have not previously had chickenpox. All children between thirteen and eighteen years of age who have not had chicken-pox should receive *two* doses of the varicella vaccine, given four to eight weeks apart.

One point about the varicella vaccine that is confusing to many parents is that the vaccine is recommended for teenagers who have "not previously been infected with varicella." But what should you do if you're not sure whether your child already had chickenpox? Some doctors recommend that if you're unsure, you should get a blood test to see if there is immunity to varicella (indicating that there was a previous chickenpox infection). However, we don't think this makes a lot of sense for two reasons. First, the blood test costs about the same as the vaccine. Second, adolescents who have already had chickenpox (and don't know it) won't be hurt by the vaccine. On the contrary, these teenagers will simply get a boost in their immunity to this virus.

For more information on the varicella vaccine, see Chapter 12.

HEPATITIS B VACCINE

The hepatitis B vaccine was recommended for all newborns in 1991. But what about the many children and teenagers who did not receive the hepatitis B vaccine at birth—should they get the vaccine?

Recommendation by the American Academy of Pediatrics

The hepatitis B vaccine is recommended to be given to all children eleven to twelve years of age. The vaccine is given as a series of three shots. The second shot is given one to two months after the first shot, and the third shot is given four to six months after the first shot.

Although the hepatitis B vaccine is now recommended for all infants born in the United States, the groups most likely to catch hepatitis B virus are teenagers and young adults. About 300,000 cases of hepatitis B virus infection occur in the United States every year, causing 10,000 hospitalizations and 400 deaths; as many as 24,000 people infected with the virus are teenagers. Therefore, it is very important to immunize children *before* they become teenagers. For this reason, the hepatitis B vaccine is recommended for all children at least by the time they are eleven to twelve years of age. In addition, we recommend that children between thirteen and eighteen years of age receive the vaccine.

Although some parents may feel that their children will never be in a group at risk for hepatitis B virus infection (see Chapter 11), about 30 to 40 percent of people who get hepatitis B virus infections are not in high-risk groups.

MEASLES-MUMPS-RUBELLA VACCINE

Severe outbreaks of measles occurred in high schools and on college campuses in the United States in the late 1980s and early 1990s—as many as 30,000 cases of measles were reported each year. Because of these outbreaks, the United States changed its policy on measles immunization in 1989. The recommendation now includes immunizing children twelve to fifteen months of age *and* again at four to six years of age. But the most important part of this change is that *all* children should have at least *two* doses of measles vaccine by the time they enter high school. This means that some children will get the second dose of the vaccine between eleven and twelve years of age.

> ## Recommendation by the American Academy of Pediatrics
>
> All children who have not received two doses of MMR vaccine are recommended to receive a second dose, preferably at eleven to twelve years of age. Those who have not received two doses by age eighteen should receive the second dose at that time.

Why did these measles outbreaks occur? Most of the teenagers and young adults infected with measles during these outbreaks had *never* received the measles vaccine; some had received the vaccine but didn't develop immunity. The requirement for a second dose of the vaccine gives many children their first chance to get it. In addition, for some children, the second dose of vaccine gives them a chance to acquire the immunity that they failed to get after the first dose. In any case, the new recommendation is working. In 1990 there were about 28,000 cases of measles reported to the Centers for Disease Control and Prevention; by 1998, there were only eighty-nine.

The second dose of mumps and rubella vaccines is given along with the measles vaccine for the reasons cited above; for many children, this is their first chance to receive the vaccines, and for others it is a chance to develop the immunity they did not develop after the first dose.

For more information on the MMR vaccine, see Chapter 10.

TETANUS-DIPHTHERIA VACCINE

Why do we need to boost the tetanus vaccine every ten years? The main reason is that immunity to tetanus fades over time. Also, teenagers and adults are always at risk for "tetanus-prone" injuries. These injuries include any puncture wounds contaminated with soil (for example, nails penetrating through sneakers). Indeed, most deaths associated with tetanus occur in adults.

> ### Recommendation by the American Academy of Pediatrics
>
> Tetanus and diphtheria vaccines (in a preparation called Td) are recommended to be given every ten years, beginning at eleven to twelve years of age.

The diphtheria vaccine is given along with the tetanus vaccine because, as with the tetanus vaccine, immunity to the diphtheria vaccine fades over time. In addition, an epidemic of diphtheria recently raged in the former Soviet Union. More than 120,000 cases, causing 4,000 deaths, occurred between 1990 and 1995. Most of those infected were not vaccinated, and most cases occurred in adults.

Diphtheria is still around in the United States. Forty-one cases and four deaths were reported between 1980 and 1995. For more information, see Chapter 7.

MENINGOCOCCUS VACCINE

Over the past two decades, several outbreaks of meningococcal infection have occurred on college campuses (see Chapter 18). For this reason, the meningococcal vaccine is recommended "to be considered" for all incoming college freshmen. The meningococcal vaccine is given as a single shot and confers excellent protection against the four types of meningococcal bacteria contained in the vaccine.

CHAPTER 34

VACCINES FOR ADULTS (INCLUDING GRANDPARENTS)

Wendy is forty years old. She takes her fifteen-year-old son to the doctor and finds out that he needs both the varicella and the hepatitis B vaccines. She is pretty sure that she has never had either chickenpox or hepatitis. Should she get these vaccines, too?

Are there any other vaccines that you need when you are an adult?

Although it may be hard to believe, every year in the United States *100 times* more adults die from vaccine-preventable diseases than children. How is this possible? First, pneumonia, caused by influenza and pneumococcus, kills 50,000 adults annually. Second, hepatitis B virus infects about 300,000 adults and kills 5,000. And third, although rare, almost all deaths caused by tetanus and diphtheria occur in adults. So whereas about 500 children die every year from diseases that are clearly preventable by vaccines, between 50,000 to 70,000 adults die from these same diseases.

Although getting vaccines is not considered by many as an adult thing to do, all adults should consider the following vaccinations for themselves.

I am forty-five years old and haven't had any shots for years. What vaccines do I need?

There are four vaccines that should be considered for use in all adults: hepatitis B, varicella, measles, and diphtheria-tetanus. Each of these vaccines is discussed below.

All adults who have not been infected with hepatitis B virus or immunized with the hepatitis B virus vaccine should get vaccinated (see Chapter 11). The vaccine is given as a series of three shots over a six-month period.

All adults who have not had a varicella infection should be vaccinated. The vaccine is given as a series of two shots over a four- to eight-week period. If one is unsure about previous infection, we recommend receiving the vaccine (see Chapter 12 for more details).

All adults born after 1956 (and, therefore, unlikely to have been naturally infected with measles virus) should receive two doses of the measles vaccine if they have not been previously immunized or infected with the virus. The vaccine should be given in the preparation called MMR, which also includes the mumps and rubella vaccines. The addition of mumps and rubella vaccines will allow for either a first-time immunization to those viruses or a boost in immunity (see Chapter 10 for more details).

Vaccines for All Adults

All adults who haven't been previously infected should be immunized with varicella, hepatitis B, tetanus-diphtheria, and measles vaccines.

Adults should receive booster doses of the tetanus and diphtheria vaccines every ten years, starting at twenty to twenty-five years of age. The vaccine is given in a preparation called Td (see Chapter 7 for more details).

I am sixty-eight years old. What vaccines do I need?

In addition to the four listed above, there are two more vaccines that should be considered for people over fifty years of age: influenza and pneumococcus.

Healthy adults over fifty years of age are at high risk of developing severe and occasionally fatal infections with influenza and pneumococcus, as compared with younger adults. For this reason, *all* adults older than fifty are recommended to receive both the pneumococcal and influenza vaccines.

Which adults need the influenza vaccine?

All adults over fifty years of age are at risk of severe pneumonia caused by influenza and should receive the influenza vaccine every year. About 90 percent of deaths from influenza occur among people older than fifty years. In addition, those at high risk of coming in contact with influenza virus should be vaccinated. This group includes doctors, nurses, and other health-care workers. Even pregnant health-care workers can be vaccinated, because the vaccine doesn't harm the fetus.

Other groups of adults are also at high risk for severe pneumonia when they get an influenza infection. For example, normal, healthy women in their third trimester of pregnancy may have a more serious case of influenza. For this reason, the Centers for Disease Control and Prevention now ask doctors to consider the influenza vaccine for all pregnant women whose third trimester falls within the influenza season (December to March). In addition, the vaccine should be used in people with long-standing heart, kidney, or lung disease (including asthma) and those with diabetes.

It should be noted that even healthy children and adults living in the same home as people at high risk of severe influenza disease should be immunized.

Which adults need the pneumococcal vaccine?

All adults over fifty years of age are at high risk of severe pneumonia caused by the pneumococcus bacteria and should, therefore, receive the pneumococcal vaccine. In addition, all adults with long-standing heart or lung disease, liver disease, alcoholism, diabetes, or cancer should receive the vaccine. The pneumonococcal vaccine that is cur-. rently given to adults is not conjugated to a protein.

Unfortunately, people who need the pneumococcal vaccine often don't receive it.

My child is in a day-care center. Are there vaccines that employees of the center should get?

It is especially important for day-care center workers to be immunized with the following vaccines: measles-mumps-rubella, tetanus-diphtheria, varicella, hepatitis B, Hib, and hepatitis A.

The hepatitis A virus is a common cause of infection in day-care centers and like, chickenpox, is much more severe in adults than children. Therefore, all adults who work in day-care centers should be immunized with the hepatitis A vaccine. This vaccine is given as a series of two shots over a six-month period (see Chapter 21).

SUMMING UP:
UNDERSTANDING
VACCINES

Fear of vaccines is not new. In 1802, the cartoonist James Gilray sketched a popular sentiment. His cartoon showed a room full of grotesque and disfigured people: their noses were snouts, their hands were hooves, and their ears were long and floppy. They were turning into cows. In the middle of the room stood a doctor holding a syringe, gazing off into the distance, disinterested. The doctor was Edward Jenner. Jenner had recently found that a cow virus (called cowpox) protected people from smallpox—a common, fatal infection. At that time, smallpox had killed more people than all other infectious diseases combined. Jenner's vaccine eventually eliminated smallpox from the face of the earth. But in the 1800s some people refused the vaccine, fearing that a virus from a cow could turn people into cows.

Today, we are amused by the ignorance and superstition of Gilray's cartoon. We are comfortable that the method, logic, and reason of science has led us into an age where we no longer believe notions as far-fetched as people turning into cows. But we're not quite as far along as we might imagine. Recently, vaccines have been blamed for diabetes, multiple sclerosis, autism, learning disabilities, violent behavior, sudden infant death syndrome, attention deficit disorder, hyperactivity, epilepsy, chronic joint disease, chronic neurologic diseases, and unexplained coma. Some parents in the United

States feel strongly that these notions are true and refuse vaccines for their children.

In this book we have tried to include the information that we hope will help parents make the best decisions for their children and themselves. We have tried to explain in a straightforward manner some fairly complex issues regarding the science, immunology, and biology of vaccines. We did this because we wanted you to understand not only the facts but also the concepts behind vaccines. We felt that this approach would best enable everyone to deal with misinformation about vaccines. Now, when people are asked to participate in decisions about vaccines, we are confident that they will be well-informed advocates for their own and their children's health.

BIBLIOGRAPHY

GENERAL SOURCES

BOOKS

Atkinson, W., Furphy, L., Gantt, J., et al., eds. *Epidemiology and Prevention of Vaccine-Preventable Diseases,* 6th ed. Centers for Disease Control and Prevention, U.S. Department of Health and Human Services, 2000.

Feigin, R. D., and Cherry, J. D., eds. *Textbook of Pediatric Infectious Diseases,* 4th ed. Philadelphia: W. B. Saunders and Co., 1998.

Humiston, Sharon, and Good, Cynthia. *Vaccinating Your Child: Questions and Answers for the Concerned Parent.* Atlanta: Peachtree Publishers Ltd., 2000. Available on the Internet at www.peachtree-online.com.

Mandell, G. L., Bennett, J. E., and Dolin, R., eds. *Principles and Practice of Infectious Diseases,* 5th ed. New York: Churchill Livingstone, 2000.

Parents' Guide to Childhood Immunization. Centers for Disease Control and Prevention, U.S. Department of Health and Human Services.

Plotkin, S. A., and Orenstein, W. A. *Vaccines,* 3rd ed. Philadelphia: W. B. Saunders and Co., 1999.

2000 Red Book: Report of Committee on Infectious Diseases, 25th ed. Elk Grove Village, Ill.: American Academy of Pediatrics, 2000.

Your Child's Best Shot: A Parent's Guide to Vaccination. Canadian Pediatric Society, Ottawa, Ontario.

Pamphlets and Other Materials

"A Parent's Guide to Childhood Immunization," "Guide to Contraindications to Childhood Vaccinations," and "Six Common Misconceptions about Vaccination," are pamphlets available from the Centers for Disease Control and Prevention (CDC) can be obtained free of charge from the CDC by calling 1-800-CDC-SHOT.

"The Facts about Childhood Vaccines," an informational tear sheet, is provided by the Vaccine Education Center at the Children's Hospital of Philadelphia and can be ordered at www.vaccine.chop.edu.

"Plain Talk about Childhood Immunizations" describes the facts behind all childhood vaccines and is offered by the Public Health Department of Seattle and King County. The pamphlet can be ordered at www.metrokc.gov/health/immunization/childimmunity.htm.

Vaccine Information Statements on all childhood and adults vaccines are offered by the Centers for Disease Control and Prevention and can be found at www.cdc.gov/nip/publications/VIS.

"Vaccines and Your Baby," a pamphlet by the Vaccine Education Center at the Children's Hospital of Philadelphia, can be ordered at www.vaccine.chop.edu or by calling 1-215-590-9990.

"General Recommendations on Immunization." *Morbidity and Mortality Weekly Report,* vol. 51, RR-2, 2002.

Videos

"Before It's Too Late, Vaccinate!," a video offered by the American Academy of Pediatrics, can be ordered by calling 1-847-981-7091.

"Vaccines and Your Baby" and "Vaccines: Separating Fact from Fear," videos available from the Vaccine Education Center at the Children's Hospital of Philadelphia, can be ordered at www.vaccine.chop.edu or by calling 1-215-590-9990.

Hotlines

Centers for Disease Control and Prevention, National Immunization Program, answers questions parents and health-care professionals have about vaccines. Information can be obtained by calling 1-800-232-2522 (English) or 800-232-0233 (Spanish) or on the Internet at www.cdc.gov/nip.

PROFESSIONAL AND PARENT GROUPS AND WEB SITES

The Albert B. Sabin Vaccine Organization is a nonprofit public organization dedicated to continuing the work of Dr. Albert Sabin, who envisioned the enormous potential of vaccines to prevent deadly diseases. The Sabin Vaccine Institute promotes rapid scientific advances in vaccine development, delivery, and distribution worldwide via vaccine research and development, academic support, and public awareness. The web site is www.sabin.org.

The Allied Vaccine Group is comprised of web sites dedicated to presenting valid scientific information about vaccines. The web site is www.vaccine.org.

The American Academy of Pediatrics (AAP) is an organization of pediatricians interested in promoting the health and well-being of children. In addition to their interest in all aspects of health care for children, the AAP has information about vaccines on their web site at www.aap.org.

Bill and Melinda Gates's Children's Vaccine Program has committed funds to support the infrastructure for vaccine delivery and education worldwide. Information can be found at www. childrensvaccine.org.

The Centers for Disease Control and Prevention offer information about vaccines on their web site at www.cdc.gov/nip.

Every Child by Two was established by the American Nurses Foundation and works to increase awareness of the need for immunizations by two years of age. The web site is www.ecbt.org.

The Immunization Action Coalition (IAC) is a nonprofit organization that works to boost immunization rates and prevent disease. The IAC provides excellent and timely information on practical tips about vaccine use and, in addition, translates vaccine information into many languages. The IAC can be found at www.immunize.org.

The Institute for Vaccine Safety is based at the Johns Hopkins Hospital and provides excellent, thorough, and up-to-date information on vaccine safety. The web site is www.vaccinesafety.edu.

The National Network for Immunization Information is a special project of the Infectious Diseases Society of America, the Pediatric Infectious Disease Society, the American Academy of Pediatrics, and the American Nurses Association. It provides excellent, up-to-date information about vaccines and vaccine safety. The web site is www.immunizationinfo.org.

Parents for Kids with Infectious Diseases (PKIDS) offers parents information about infectious diseases and provides support services for parents of children with long-term infections (such as hepatitis B virus). The web site is www.pkids.org.

The Vaccine Education Center at the Children's Hospital of Philadelphia is composed of scientists, mothers, and fathers interested in explaining the science of vaccines in a clear and straightforward manner. The web site is www.vaccine.chop.edu.

The Vaccine Page is a source of daily news on vaccines from multiple sources. The web site is www.vaccines.org.

TEXT SOURCES

HOW ARE VACCINES MADE?

The story of mumps

Buynak, E. B., and Hilleman, M. R. "Live attenuated mumps virus vaccine. I. Vaccine development." *Proceedings of the Society of Experimental Biology and Medicine,* vol. 123, pp. 768–775, 1966.

Hilleman, M. R., Buynak, E. B., Weibel, R. E., and Stokes, J., Jr. "Live, attenuated mumps-virus vaccine." *New England Journal of Medicine,* vol. 278, pp. 227–232, 1968.

Interview with Maurice Hilleman on December 3, 1996. West Point, PA.

"Mumps vaccine: Recommendation of the Public Health Service Advisory Committee on Immunization Practices." *Morbidity and Mortality Weekly Report,* vol. 26, pp. 393–394, 1977.

Pagano, J. S., Levine, R. H., Sugg, W. C., and Finger, J. A. "Clinical trial of new attenuated mumps virus vaccine (Jeryl Lynn Strain): preliminary report." *Progress in Immunobiologic Standardization,* vol. 3, pp. 196–202. New York: Karger, Basel, 1969.

The Cutter incident

Hinman, A. R., and Thacker, S. B. Invited commentary on "The Cutter incident: Poliomyelitis following formaldehyde-inactivated poliovirus vaccination in the United States during the spring of 1955. II. Relationship of poliomyelitis to Cutter vaccine." *American Journal of Epidemiology,* vol. 142, pp. 107–108, 1995.

Nathanson, N., and Langmuir, A. D. "The Cutter incident: Poliomyelitis following formaldehyde-inactivated poliovirus vaccination in the United States during the spring of 1955. I. Background." *American Journal of Hygiene,* vol. 78, pp. 16–28, 1963.

Nathanson, N., and Langmuir, A. D. "The Cutter incident: Poliomyelitis following formaldehyde-inactivated poliovirus vaccination in the United States during the spring of 1955. II. Relationship of poliomyelitis to Cutter vaccine." *American Journal of Hygiene,* vol. 78, pp. 16–28, 1963.

The story of the RSV vaccine

Chin, J., Magoffin, R. L., Shearer, L. A., et al. "Field evaluation of a respiratory syncytial vaccine and a trivalent parainfluenza virus vaccine in a pediatric population." *American Journal of Epidemiology,* vol. 89, pp. 449–463, 1969.

Fulginiti, V. A., Eller, J. J., Sieber, O. F., et al. "Respiratory virus immunization. I. A field trial of two inactivated respiratory virus vaccines; an aqueous trivalent parainfluenza virus vaccine and an alum-precipitated respiratory syncytial virus vaccine." *American Journal of Epidemiology,* vol. 89, pp. 435–448, 1969.

Kapikian, A. Z., Mitchell, R. H., Chanock, R. M., et al. "An epidemiologic study of altered clinical reactivity to respiratory syncytial (RS) virus infection in children previously vaccinated with inactivated RS virus vaccine." *American Journal of Epidemiology,* vol. 89, pp. 405–421, 1969.

Kim, H. W., Canchola, J. G., Brandt, C. D., et al. "Respiratory syncytial virus disease in infants despite prior administration of antigen inactivated vaccine." *American Journal of Epidemiology,* vol. 89, pp. 422–434, 1969.

Piedra, P. A., Hiatt, P. W., Grace, S., et al. "Safety and efficacy of PFP-2 vaccine during respiratory syncytial virus season in children with cystic fibrosis." Presented at the 36th Interscience Conference on Antimicrobial Agents and Chemotherapy, New Orleans. September 15–18, 1996. Abstract H50.

ARE VACCINES SAFE?

Baker, S. P. *The Injury Fact Book.* Lexington, Mass.: Lexington Books, 1984.

Budnick, L. D., and Ross, D. A. "Bathtub-related drownings in the United States, 1979–1981." *American Journal of Public Health,* vol. 75, pp. 630–633, 1985.

Dingle, J. G., Badger, G. F., and Jordan, W. S. *Illness in the Home: A Study of 25,000 Illnesses in a Group of Cleveland Families.* Cleveland: The Press of Western Reserve University, 1964.

Duclos, P. J., and Sanderson, L. M. "An epidemiological description of lightning-related deaths in the United States." *International Journal of Epidemiology,* vol. 19, pp. 673–679, 1990.

Howson, C. P., Howe, C. J., and Fineberg, H. V., eds. *Adverse Effects of Pertussis and Rubella Vaccines.* Washington, D.C.: National Academy Press, 1991.

Ross, J. F. "Risk: Where do real dangers lie?" *Smithsonian,* November 1995.

Stratton, K. R., Howe, C. J., and Johnston, R. B., Jr., eds. *Adverse Events Associated with Childhood Vaccines: Evidence Bearing on Causality.* Washington, D.C.: National Academy Press, 1994.

"Update: Vaccine side effects, adverse reactions, contraindications, and precautions." *Morbidity and Mortality Weekly Report,* vol. 45, September 6, 1996.

WHO RECOMMENDS VACCINES?

"Recommended childhood immunization schedule—United States, 2002." Centers for Disease Control and Prevention.

Title 28, Part III, Chapter 23, Subchapter C of the Commonwealth of Pennsylvania's School Health Immunization Legislation.

DTaP

Committee on Infectious Diseases of the American Academy of Pediatrics. "Acellular pertussis vaccine: Recommendations for use as the initial series in infants and children." *Pediatrics,* vol. 99, pp. 282–288, 1997.

Greco, D., Salmaso, S., Mastrantonio, P., et al. "A controlled trial of two acellular vaccines and one whole-cell vaccine against pertussis." *New England Journal of Medicine,* vol. 334, pp. 341–348, 1996.

Griffin, M. R., Ray, W. A., Livengood, J. R., et al. "Risk of sudden infant death syndrome after immunization with the diphtheria-tetanus-pertussis vaccine." *New England Journal of Medicine,* vol. 319, pp. 618–623, 1988.

Howson, C. P., and Fineberg, H. V. "Adverse events following pertussis and rubella vaccines: Summary of a report of the Institute of Medicine." *Journal of the American Medical Association,* vol. 267, pp. 392–396, 1992.

Rock, A. "The lethal dangers of the billion-dollar vaccine business." *Money,* pp. 148–164, December 1996.

"Update: Vaccine side effects, adverse reactions, contraindications, and precautions." *Morbidity and Mortality Weekly Report,* vol. 45, September 6, 1996.

Wortis, N., Strebel, P. M., Wharton, M., et al. "Pertussis deaths: Report of 23 cases in the United States, 1992–1993." *Pediatrics,* vol. 97, pp. 607–612, 1996.

POLIO

Black, K. *In the Shadow of Polio: A Personal and Social History.* Boston: Addison-Wesley Publishing Co., 1996.

Faden, H., Modlin, J. F., Thoms, M. L., et al. "Comparative evaluation of immunization with live attenuated and enhanced-potency inactivated trivalent poliovirus vaccines in childhood: Systemic and local immune responses." *Journal of Infectious Diseases,* vol. 162, pp. 1291–1297, 1990.

Judelsohn, R. "Changing the US polio immunization schedule would be bad public health policy." *Pediatrics,* vol. 98, pp. 115–116, 1996.

Katz, S. "Poliovirus policy—time for a change." *Pediatrics,* vol. 98, pp. 116–117, 1996.

Nkowane, B. M., Wassilak, S. G. F., Orenstein, W. A., et al. "Vaccine-associated paralytic poliomyelitis." *Journal of the American Medical Association,* vol. 257, pp. 1335–1340, 1987.

Paradiso, P. R. "The future of polio immunization in the United States: Are we ready for a change?" *Pediatric Infectious Disease Journal,* vol. 15, pp. 645–649, 1996.

Plotkin, S. A. "Inactivated polio vaccine for the United States: A missed vaccination opportunity." *Pediatric Infectious Diseases Journal,* vol. 14, pp. 835–839, 1995.

HIB

"Recommendations for use of Haemophilus b conjugate vaccines and a combined diphtheria, tetanus, pertussis, and Haemophilus influenzae type b vaccine." *Morbidity and Mortality Weekly Report,* vol. 42, September 17, 1993.

MMR

Measles

Davis, S. F., Strebel, P. M., Atkinson, W. L., et al. "Reporting efficiency during a measles outbreak in New York City, 1991." *American Journal of Public Health,* vol. 83, pp. 1011–1015, 1993.

James, J. M., Burks, A. W., Robertson, P. K., and Sampson, H. A. "Safe administration of the measles vaccine to children allergic to eggs." *New England Journal of Medicine,* vol. 332, pp. 1262–1266, 1995.

"Update: Vaccine side effects, adverse reactions, contraindications, and precautions." *Morbidity and Mortality Weekly Report,* vol. 45, September 6, 1996.

Watson, J. C., Pearson, J. A., Markowitz, L. E., et al. "An evaluation of measles revaccination among school-entry aged children." *Pediatrics,* vol. 97, pp. 613–618, 1996.

Wicks, S. *History of Medicine in New Jersey.* Newark, N.J.: M. R. Dennis and Co., 1879.

Mumps

Hilleman, M. R. "Past, present and future of measles, mumps, and rubella virus vaccines." *Pediatrics,* vol. 90, pp. 149–153, 1992.

"Update: Vaccine side effects, adverse reactions, contraindications, and precautions." *Morbidity and Mortality Weekly Report,* vol. 45, September 6, 1996.

Rubella

Fulginiti, V. A. "How safe are the pertussis and rubella vaccines? A commentary on the Institute of Medicine report." *Pediatrics,* vol. 89, pp. 334–336, 1992.

Gregg, N. M. "Congenital cataract following German measles in the mother." *Transactions of the Ophthalmologic Society of Australia,* vol. 3, pp. 35–46, 1941.

Howson, C. P., and Fineberg, H. V. "The ricochet of magic bullets: Summary of the Institute of Medicine report, Adverse effects of pertussis and rubella vaccines." *Pediatrics,* vol. 89, pp. 318–324, 1992.

HEPATITIS B

Dienstag, J. L. "Toward the control of hepatitis B." *New England Journal of Medicine,* vol. 303, pp. 875–876, 1980.

"Hepatitis B virus: A comprehensive strategy for eliminating transmission in the United States through universal childhood vaccination." Recommendations of the Immunization Practices Advisory Committee (ACIP). *Morbidity and Mortality Weekly Report,* vol. 40, November 22, 1991.

Mulley, A. G., Silverstein, M. D., and Dienstag, J. L. "Indications for use of hepatitis B vaccine, based on cost-effectiveness analysis." *New England Journal of Medicine,* vol. 307, pp. 644–652, 1982.

Muraskin, W. *The war against hepatitis B: A history of the international task force on hepatitis B immunization.* Philadelphia: University of Pennsylvania Press, 1995.

Szmuness, W., Stevens, C. E., Harley, E. J., et al. "Hepatitis B vaccine: Demonstration of efficacy in a controlled clinical trial in a high-risk population in the United States." *New England Journal of Medicine,* vol. 303, pp. 833–841, 1980.

"Universal hepatitis B immunization." *Pediatrics,* vol. 89, pp. 795–800, 1992.

"Update: Vaccine side effects, adverse reactions, contraindications, and precautions." *Morbidity and Mortality Weekly Report,* vol. 45, September 6, 1996.

VARICELLA

Asano, Y., Suga, S., Yoshikawa, T., et al. "Experience and reason: Twenty-year follow-up of protective immunity of the Oka strain live varicella vaccine." *Pediatrics,* vol. 94, pp. 524–526, 1994.

Doctor, A., Harper, M. B., and Fleisher, G. R. "Group A β-hemolytic streptococcal bacteremia: Historical overview, changing incidence, and recent association with varicella." *Pediatrics,* vol. 96, pp. 428–433, 1995.

Fleisher, G., Henry, W., McSorley, M., et al. "Life-threatening complications of varicella." *American Journal of Diseases in Children,* vol. 135, pp. 896–899, 1981.

Hardy, I., Gershon, A. A., Steinberg, S. P., et al. "The incidence of zoster after immunization with live attenuated varicella vaccine: A study in children with leukemia." *New England Journal of Medicine,* vol. 325, pp. 1545–1550, 1991.

Pastuszak, A. L., Levy, M., Schick, B., et al. "Outcome after maternal varicella infection in the first 20 weeks of pregnancy." *New England Journal of Medicine,* vol. 330, pp. 901–905, 1994.

Plotkin, S. A. "Varicella vaccine." *Pediatrics,* vol. 97, pp. 251–253, 1996.

"Recommendations for the use of live attenuated varicella vaccine." *Pediatrics,* vol. 95, pp. 791–796, 1995.

Weibel, R. E., Neff, B. J., Kuter, B. J., et al. "Live, attenuated varicella virus vaccine: Efficacy trial in healthy children." *New England Journal of Medicine,* vol. 310, pp. 1409–1415, 1984.

PRACTICAL TIPS ABOUT VACCINES

Dennehy, P. H., Saracen, C. L., and Peter, G. "Seroconversion rates to combined measles-mumps-rubella-varicella vaccine of children with upper respiratory tract infection." *Pediatrics,* vol. 94, pp. 514–516, 1994.

French, G. M., Painter, E. C., and Coury, D. L. "Blowing away shot pain: A technique for pain management during immunization." *Pediatrics,* vol. 93, pp. 384–388, 1994.

Halsey, N. A., Boulos, R., Mode, F., et al. "Response to measles vaccine in Haitian infants 6 to 12 months old: Influence of maternal antibodies, malnutrition, and concurrent illness." *New England Journal of Medicine,* vol. 313, pp. 544–549, 1985.

King, G. E., Markowitz, L. E., Heath, J., et al. "Antibody response to measles-mumps-rubella vaccine of children with mild illness at the time of vaccination." *Journal of the American Medical Association,* vol. 275, pp. 704–707, 1996.

Ndikuyeze, A., Munoz, A., Stewart, J., et al. "Immunogenicity and safety of measles vaccine in ill African children." *International Journal of Epidemiology,* vol. 17, pp. 448–455, 1988.

Peter, G., ed. *1997 Red Book: Report of the Committee on Infectious Diseases,* 24th ed. Elk Grove Village, Ill.: American Academy of Pediatrics, 1997.

Ratnam, S., West, R., and Gadag, V. "Measles and rubella antibody response after measles-mumps-rubella vaccination in children with afebrile upper respiratory tract infection." *Journal of Pediatrics,* vol. 127, pp. 432–434, 1995.

COMMON CONCERNS ABOUT VACCINES

Adrien, J., et al. "Autism and family home movies: Preliminary findings." *Journal of Autism and Developmental Disorders,* vol. 21, pp. 43–49, 1991.

Adrien, J., et al. "Early symptoms in autism from family home movies: Evaluation and comparison between 1st and 2nd year of life using I.B.S.E. scale." *Acta Paedopsychiatrica,* vol. 55, pp. 71–75, 1992.

Ascherio, A., Zhang, S., Hernan, M., et al. "Hepatitis b vaccination and the risk of multiple sclerosis." *New England Journal of Medicine,* vol. 344, pp. 327–332, 2001.

Black, S. B., Cherry, J. D., Shinefield, H. R., et al. "Apparent decreased risk of invasive bacterial disease after heterologous childhood immunization." *American Journal of Diseases of Children,* vol. 145, pp. 746–749, 1991.

Carbone, M., Pass, H. I., Rizzo, P., et al. "Simian virus 40-like DNA sequences in human pleural mesothelioma." *Oncogene,* vol. 9, pp. 1781–1790, 1994.

Carbone, M., Rizzo, P., Procopic, A., et al. "SV40-like sequences in human bone tumors." *Oncogene,* vol. 13, pp. 527–535, 1996.

Chess, S. "Autism in children with congenital rubella." *Journal of Autism and Childhood Schizophrenia,* vol. 1, pp. 33–47, 1971.

Chess, S., Fernandez, P., and Korn, S. "Behavioral consequences of congenital rubella." *Journal of Pediatrics,* vol. 93, pp. 699–703, 1978.

Cohn, M., and Langman, R. E. "The Protecton: The unit of humoral immunity selected by evolution." *Immunological Reviews,* vol. 115, pp. 11–147, 1990.

Confavreux, C., Suissa, S., Saddier, P., et al. "Vaccinations and the relative risk of relapse in multiple sclerosis." *New England Journal of Medicine,* vol. 344, pp. 319–326, 2001.

Curtis, T. "The Origin of AIDS: A startling new theory attempts to answer the question 'Was it an act of God or an act of man?'" *Rolling Stone,* March 19, 1992.

Dales, L., et al. "Time trends in autism and in MMR immunization coverage in California." *Journal of the American Medical Association,* vol. 285, pp. 1183–1185, 2001.

Davidson, M., Letson, W., Ward, J. I., et al. "DTP immunization and susceptibility to infectious diseases. Is there a relationship?" *American Journal of Diseases of Children,* vol. 145, pp. 750–754, 1991.

DeStefano, F., Mullooly, J. P., Okoro, C. A., et al. "Childhood vaccinations, vaccination timing, and risk of type 1 diabetes mellitus." *Pediatrics,* vol. 108, p. E112, 2001.

Deykin, E.Y., and MacMahon, B. "Viral exposure and autism." *American Journal of Epidemiology,* vol. 109, pp. 628–638, 1979.

Feldman, R. B., Pinsky, L., Mendelson, J., and Lajoie, R. "Can language disorder not due to peripheral deafness be an isolated expression of prenatal rubella?" *Pediatrics,* vol. 52, pp. 296–299, 1973.

Feldman, R. B., Lajoie, R., Mendelson, J., and Pinsky, L. "Congenital rubella and language disorders." *Lancet,* vol. 2, p. 978, 1971.

Garrett, A. J., Dunham, A., and Wood, D. J. "Retroviruses and polio vaccines." *Lancet,* pp. 932–933, October 9, 1993.

Halsey, N.A., et al. "Hepatitis B vaccine and central nervous system demyelinating diseases." *Pediatric Infectious Disease Journal,* vol. 18, pp. 23–24, 1999.

The Institute for Vaccine Safety Diabetes Workshop Panel. "Childhood immunizations and type 1 diabetes: Summary of an Institute for Vaccine Safety Workshop." *Pediatric Infectious Disease Journal,* vol. 18, pp. 217–222, 1999.

Kaye, J. A., et al. "Mumps, measles, and rubella vaccine and the incidence of autism recorded by general practitioners: A time trend analysis." *British Medical Journal,* vol. 322, pp. 460–463, 2001.

Khan, A. S., Shahabuddin, M., Bryan, T., et al. "Analysis of live, oral poliovirus vaccine monopools for human immunodeficiency virus type 1 and simian immunodeficiency virus." *Journal of Infectious Diseases,* vol. 174, pp. 1185–1190, 1996.

Lubinsky, M. "Behavioral consequences of congenital rubella." *Journal of Pediatrics,* vol. 94, pp. 678–679, 1979.

Mars, A.J., et al. "Symptoms of pervasive developmental disorders as observed in prediagnostic home videos of infants and toddlers." *Journal of Pediatrics,* vol. 132, pp. 500–504, 1998.

Madsen, K. M., Hvid, A., Vestergaard, M., et al. " A population-based study of measles, mumps, and rubella vaccination and autism." *New England Journal of Medicine,* vol. 347, pp. 1477–1482, 2002.

Miller, N. Z. *Vaccines: Are They Really Safe and Effective?* Santa Fe, N.M.: New Atlantean Press, 1996.

Neustaedter, R. *The Vaccine Guide: Making an Informed Choice.* Berkeley, Calif.: North Atlantic Books, 1996.

Offit, P. A., Quarles, J., Gerber, M. A., et al. "Addressing parents' concerns: Do multiple vaccines overwhelm or weaken the infant's immune system?" *Pediatrics,* vol. 109, pp. 124–129, 2002.

Osterling, J., et al. "Early recognition of children with autism: A study of first birthday home videotapes." *Journal of Autism and Developmental Disorders,* vol. 24, pp. 247–257, 1994.

Otto, S., Mahner, B., Kadow, I, et al. "General non-specific morbidity is reduced after vaccination within the third month of life—the Greifswald study." *Journal of Infection,* vol. 41, pp. 172–175, 2000.

Rock, A. "The lethal dangers of the billion-dollar vaccine business." *Money,* pp. 148–164, December 1996.

Rodier P., et al. "Embryological origin for autism: Developmental anomalies of the cranial nerve motor nuclei." *Journal of Comparative Neurology,* vol. 370, pp. 247–261, 1996.

Storsaeter, J., Olin, P., Renemar, B., et al. "Mortality and morbidity from invasive bacterial infections during a clinical trial of acellular pertussis vaccines in Sweden." *Pediatric Infectious Diseases Journal,* vol. 7, pp. 637–645, 1988.

Stromland, K., et al. "Autism in thalidomide embropathy: A population study." *Developmental Medicine and Child Neurology,* vol. 36, pp. 351–356, 1994.

Swisher, C. N., and Swisher, L. "Congenital rubella and autistic behavior." *New England Journal of Medicine,* vol. 293, p. 198, 1975.

Taylor, B., et al. "Autism and measles, mumps, and rubella vaccine: No epidemiological evidence for a causal association." *Lancet,* vol. 353, pp. 2026–2029, 1999.

Taylor, B., et al. "Measles, mumps, and rubella vaccination and bowel problems or developmental regression in children with autism: Population study." *British Medical Journal,* vol. 324, pp. 393–396, 2002.

Teitelbaum, P., et al. "Movement analysis in infancy may be useful for the early diagnosis of autism." *Proceedings of the National Academy of Sciences USA,* vol. 95, pp. 13982–13987, 1998.

Uhlmann, V., et al. "Potential viral pathogenic mechanism for new variant inflammatory bowel disease." *Journal of Clinical Pathology: Molecular Pathology,* vol. 55, pp. 1–6, 2002.

"Vaccination: The issue of our times." In *Mothering: The Magazine of Natural Family Living,* no. 79, pp. 26–80, Summer 1996.

Wakefield, A. J., et al. "Ileal-lymphoid-nodular hyperplasia, non-specific colitis, and pervasive developmental disorder in children." *Lancet,* vol. 351, pp. 637–641, 1998.

Wechsler, P. "A Shot in the Dark." *New York,* pp. 39–85, November 11, 1996.

RABIES

de Kruif, P. *Microbe Hunters.* New York: Harcourt, Brace and Co., 1926.

Fishbein, D. B., and Robinson, L. E. "Rabies." *New England Journal of Medicine,* vol. 329, pp. 1632–1638, 1993.

INFLUENZA

Asbury, A. K. "The swine flu incident revisited." *Annals of Neurology,* vol. 16, pp. 513–514, 1984.

Beghi, E., Kurland, L. T., Mulder, D. W., and Wiederholt, W. C. "Guillain-Barré syndrome: Clinicoepidemiologic features and effect of influenza vaccine." *Archives of Neurology,* vol. 42, pp. 1053–1057, 1985.

Hoehling, A. A. *The Great Epidemic.* Boston: Little Brown and Co., 1961.

Lasky, T., Terracciano, G., Magder, L., et al. "Guillain-Barré syndrome and the 1992–1993 and 1993–1994 influenza vaccines." *New England Journal of Medicine,* vol. 339, pp. 1797–1802, 1998.

Murphy, K. R., and Strunk, R. C. "Safe administration of influenza vaccine in asthmatic children hypersensitive to egg proteins." *Journal of Pediatrics,* vol. 106, pp. 931–933, 1985.

"Prevention and control of influenza: Recommendations of the Advisory Committee on Immunization Practices (ACIP)." *Morbidity and Mortality Weekly Report,* vol. 45, May 3, 1996.

Reichert, T. A., Sugya, N., Fedson, D., et al. "The Japanese experience with vaccinating schoolchildren against influenza." *New England Journal of Medicine,* vol. 344, pp. 889–896, 2001.

Safranek, T. J., Lawrence, D. N., Kurland, L. T., et al. "Reassessment of the association between Guillain-Barré syndrome and receipt of swine influenza vaccine in 1976–1977: Results of a two-state study." *American Journal of Epidemiology,* vol. 133, pp. 940–951, 1991.

Wade, N. "1976 swine flu campaign faulted yet principals would do it again." *Science,* vol. 202, pp. 849–852, 1978.

Lyme

Gross, D. M., Forsthuber, T., Tary-Lehmann, M., et al. "Identification of LFA-1 as a candidate autoantigen in treatment-resistant Lyme arthritis." *Science,* vol. 281, pp. 703–706, 1998.

Lathrop, S. "Adverse event reports following vaccination for Lyme disease: December 1998–July 2000." *Vaccine,* vol. 20, pp. 1603–1608, 2002.

Tuberculosis

Bates, J. H., and Stead, W. W. "The history of tuberculosis as a global epidemic." *Medical Clinics of North America,* vol. 77, pp. 1205–1217, 1993.

Grange, J. M., Gibson, J., Osborn, T. W., et al. "What is BCG?" *Tubercle,* vol. 64, pp. 129–139, 1983.

Houk, V. H., Kent, D. C., Baker, J. H., et al. "The Byrd study: In-depth analysis of a micro-outbreak of tuberculosis in a closed environment." *Archives of Environmental Health,* vol. 16, pp. 4–6, 1968.

"The role of BCG vaccine in the prevention and control of tuberculosis in the United States: A joint statement by the Advisory Council for the Elimination of Tuberculosis and the Advisory Committee on Immunization Practices." *Morbidity and Mortality Weekly Report,* vol. 45, April 26, 1996.

Stead, W. W. "Tuberculosis among elderly persons: An outbreak in a nursing home." *Annals of Internal Medicine,* vol. 94, pp. 606–610, 1981.

SOURCES OF INFORMATION ABOUT VACCINES FOR TRAVELERS

"Health Information for International Travel 1999–2000." U.S. Department of Health and Human Services, Centers for Disease Control and Prevention, National Center for Infectious Diseases, Atlanta, Georgia.

Wade, B. "Finding out about vaccines." *New York Times,* November 24, 1996.

HEPATITIS A

Koff, R.S. "The case for routine childhood vacination against hepatitis A." *New England Journal of Medicine,* vol. 340, pp. 644–645, 1999.

"Licensure of inactivated hepatitis A vaccine and recommendations for use among international travelers." *Morbidity and Mortality Weekly Report,* vol. 44, pp. 559–560, 1995.

Margolis, H. S., and Alter, M. J. "Will hepatitis A become a vaccine-preventable disease?" *Annals of Internal Medicine,* vol. 122, pp. 464–465, 1995.

CHOLERA

Mann, T. *Death in Venice.* New York: Alfred A. Knopf, 1930.

"Recommendation of the Immunization Practices Advisory Committee (ACIP): Cholera vaccine." *Morbidity and Mortality Weekly Report,* vol. 37, pp. 617–624, 1988.

TYPHOID

"Typhoid immunization: Recommendations of the Advisory Committee on Immunization Practices (ACIP)." *Morbidity and Mortality Weekly Report,* vol. 43, December 9, 1994.

Japanese Encephalitis Virus

"Inactivated Japanese encephalitis virus vaccine: Recommendations of the Advisory Committee on Immunization Practices (ACIP)." *Morbidity and Mortality Weekly Report,* vol. 42, January 8, 1993.

RSV

Committee on Infectious Diseases, Committee on Fetus and Newborn, American Academy of Pediatrics. "Respiratory syncytial virus immune globulin intravenous: Indications for use." *Pediatrics,* vol. 99, pp. 645–650, 1997.

Piedra, P. A., Hiatt, P. W., Grace, S., et al. "Safety and efficacy of PFP-2 vaccine during respiratory syncytial virus season in children with cystic fibrosis." Presented at the 36th Interscience Conference on Antimicrobial Agents and Chemotherapy, New Orleans. September 15–18, 1996. Abstract H50.

Rodriguez, W. J., Gruber, W. C., Welliver, R. C., et al. "Respiratory syncytial virus (RSV) immune globulin intravenous therapy for RSV lower respiratory tract infection in infants and young children at high risk for severe RSV infections." *Pediatrics,* vol. 99, pp. 454–461, 1997.

Smallpox

Cohen, J. "Smallpox vaccinations: How much protection remains?" *Science,* vol. 294, page 885, 2001.

Vaccines for Adults

Gardner, P., and Schaffner, W. "Immunization of adults." *New England Journal of Medicine,* vol. 328, pp. 1252–1258, 1993.

"Update on adult immunization: Recommendations of the Immunization Practices Advisory Subcommittee (ACIP)." *Morbidity and Mortality Weekly Report,* vol. 40, November 15, 1991.

INDEX

231

About the Authors

Paul A. Offit

Dr. Offit is chief of the Division of Infectious Diseases and the Henle Professor of Immunologic and Infectious Diseases at the Children's Hospital of Philadelphia and Professor of Pediatrics at the University of Pennsylvania School of Medicine. He is the recipient of a number of awards including the J. Edmund Bradley Prize for Excellence in Pediatrics, the Young Investigator Award in Vaccine Development, and the University of Pennsylvania Research Foundation Award. He is an internationally recognized expert in the fields of immunology and virology. He is also, with Bonnie Fass-Offit and Louis Bell, the coauthor of a book entitled *Breaking the Antibiotic Habit: A Parent's Guide to Coughs, Colds, Ear Infections, and Sore Throats.*

Louis M. Bell

Dr. Bell is chief of the Division of General Pediatrics at the Children's Hospital of Philadelphia and Professor of Pediatrics at the University of Pennsylvania School of Medicine. He is the recipient of many awards, including an outstanding achievement award in early childhood immunization presented by the U.S. Secretary of Health and Human Services and the Dean's Award from the University of Pennsylvania School of Medicine for excellence in clinical teaching. He is also the recipient of a grant from the Centers for Disease Control and Prevention to enhance preschool immunizations and served as cochair of the West Philadelphia Immunization Project.